Treating Intellectually Disabled Sex Offenders

A Model Residential Program

James Haaven, M.A.
Roger Little, M.S.
Dan Petre-Miller, M.S.

The Safer Society Press
Shoreham Depot Road
RR1, Box 24-B
Orwell, VT 05760-9756
802-897-7541

Library of Congress Catalog Card #89-63433

Cover Design: Theresa McCloud

Photos: James Haaven

Editors: Euan Bear, Fay Honey Knopp, & Lois B. Lackey

The publisher and authors thank the following for permission to quote from or adapt copyrighted material: Paul H. Brookes Publishing for *Changing Inappropriate Sexual Behavior: A Community-based Approach for Persons with Developmental Disabilities* by Dorothy Griffiths, Vernon Quinsey, & David Hingsburger / William D. Pithers for the diagram, "A cognitive/behavioral model of the relapse process." From Pithers, W.D., Kashima, K.M., Cumming, G.F., Beal, L.S., & Buell, M.M. (1988). Relapse prevention of sexual aggression. In R.A. Prentky & V.R. Quinsey (Eds.). *Human sexual aggression: Current perspectives.* Annals of the New York Academy of Sciences: Vol. 528 (p. 248). New York: The New York Academy of Sciences.

Order from:

The Safer Society Press
Shoreham Depot Road
RR1, Box 24-B
Orwell, VT 05760-9756
802-897-7541

$24.00 / Single copy price includes postage & handling

ALL ORDERS MUST BE PREPAID, U.S. FUNDS ONLY
Vermont residents, please add sales tax

Authors' Acknowledgments

Ten years ago it was a very bold step to initiate a treatment opportunity for the intellectually disabled offender who so often "falls through the cracks" of the mental health system. We are grateful for the vision of the initial task force, chaired by Deputy Director of Corrections Thomas Toombs, and the Oregon Legislature, spearheaded by Representative Vera Katz and Senator Fred Heard, which created the Social Skills Program. Since the Program's inception, the Mental Health Division and Corrections Department have continually worked in a cooperative and creative way to provide us with direction and support.

For their consistent and unwavering assistance and confidence, we also sincerely thank those from other agencies and friends in the community who have contributed so much to our work here.

We hope this book will prove useful in helping to advance the technology of sex-offender treatment for the intellectually disabled. We also hope it will serve to reinforce the possibility of effectively working with this unique population and the importance of continuing that work.

Special Acknowledgments

Elaine Ferguson
Roger Smith
Gerry Warren
Velma Fidler
Gordon Bradford
Elaine Roper
Ilene Whelden
Eileen Lundquist
Don Barrows
William Bennett
Don Ventres
Bob Polen
John Priollaud
Charles Faulk
Tom Masters
Bruce Stock
Debi Cedarburg
Stan Brown
Kathleen Davis
Gene Luffman
Michael McNamara
Eicca Smith
Yvonne Hendricks

Publisher's Acknowledgments

The Safer Society Press thanks Emily Coleman, Michael Comte, Georgia Cumming, Robert Freeman-Longo, and Kathy Kaufman for reading and commenting on this manuscript, and Douglas Biklen for his comments and advice.

Funding in part for this publication was provided through a grant to the Ohio Youth Services Network from the Ohio Governor's Office of Criminal Justice Services.

Foreword

Although it was more than 15 years ago, I remember clearly the first intellectually disabled sex-offender client I treated. Unfortunately, my first sight of him raised my own prejudiced, stereotyped, and uneducated notions. I saw him as a Humpty Dumpty figure in worn denim bib overalls. His halting speech and withdrawn style further fed my bias. I thought, "He can't help himself. How can he learn not to touch children?" This attitude, still so common, obviously does this population a grave injustice by belittling them as people, absolving them of responsibility, and incorrectly assuming treatment will not be effective.

In the process of working with this client, I learned of his brave struggle to face his sexual problem in spite of the denial of his family and the reluctance and inability of many mental health professionals to deal with him. I came to see him as a dignified person who deserved the quality treatment he wanted, needed, and could use.

Although I recognized the need for quality treatment, I was still unclear how to proceed clinically. Basic information about the characteristics of this population and related adjustments in assessment and treatment approaches was lacking, a situation that is gradually changing. A 1980 survey of residential facilities serving intellectually disabled clients throughout the United States indicated that only 10 of the 131 respondents knew of any in-state programs serving these types of sex offenders (Coleman & Murphy, 1980, p. 272). Eight years later, a survey conducted by The Safer Society Program revealed that 169 adult and 222 adolescent programs offer some kind of specialized services. This increase in the availability of services is an indication of growing awareness.

However, the pressing need for knowledge about this population far exceeds the gains we've made. *Treating Intellectually Disabled Sex Offenders: A Model Residential Program* helps considerably in lessening this gap. It provides both the nuts-and-bolts technology and the treatment philosophy needed to work with this neglected population. The authors describe in a clear and practical manner a well established comprehensive and effective program. Mental health practitioners and administrators will find it invaluable in developing and/or augmenting treatment programs for their own populations. The concepts and approaches can be adapted to outpatient programs and to different staff/client ratios as well.

Legal professionals and advocates for the intellectually disabled can also benefit from the message inherent throughout the book: that intellectually disabled sex offenders should be held accountable for their actions and can learn to gain control of their sexual problems and reshape their lives.

The authors demonstrate a realistic appreciation of the depth and intricacies of the challenges posed by this unique group of clients. They simultaneously encourage and teach perseverance and skills needed to face these difficulties. I wish I had this book so many years ago when I initially struggled with my own bias and ignorance toward that first intellectually disabled sex-offender client. I also wish he had had the opportunity to participate in a program like the Social Skills Program at Oregon State Hospital. Fortunately many others, perhaps also previously seen as hopeless Humpty Dumpty figures, can now be perceived accurately through the solid clinical information offered in this wonderful book. I feel doubly grateful now to have such a book available to all of us. It has much to offer both the beginner and the seasoned practitioner. The authors have provided a heartening blend of specific techniques with hope and respect for the clients we serve and the work we do.

Emily Coleman, M.A.
Director, Sex Offender Program
Franklin County Mental Health Center
Greenfield, MA

TABLE OF CONTENTS

PART I

BACKGROUND

INTRODUCTION

Treating Intellectually Disabled Sex Offenders: A Model Residential Program addresses the needs of a population embodying two issues society would prefer to ignore: the potential for persons identified as "intellectually disabled" to change their thoughts and behaviors, and the treatability of sex offenders. Authors James Haaven, Roger Little, and Dan Petre-Miller know from experience that intellectually disabled sex offenders can be taught to survive offense-free in the wider community.

In the last few decades, society has begun to understand that disabled persons have the potential to "normalize" their lives.[1] Likewise, strides have been made in demonstrating that sex offenders have the potential to learn to control their aggressive behaviors (Knopp, 1984). Despite these gains, societal confusion continues to surround these two concepts.

The confusion begins with how society thinks about intellectually disabled people as *sexual* persons. On one hand they are perceived as asexual, "holy innocents," perpetual infants; on the other as "oversexed"[2] and dangerous.[3] An understanding of basic patterns of male sexual behavior[4] *in general* may help advocates and agency personnel comprehend the relevance and necessity of certain types of interventions into maladaptive sexual behaviors. Though more complex when intellectually disabled sex offenders are involved, principles such as the following six (adapted from

---

[1] See Biklen (1989): "Happily, this sought after social condition is not just a vision. There are two areas of people's lives in which the experience of ordinariness is now occasionally achieved. These areas are self-definition and family relationships. In a third area, namely social institutions (e.g., schools), unconditional inclusion has been more difficult, though not without some emerging form" (p. 1).

[2] See Griffiths, Quinsey, & Hingsburger (1989): "People still believe that [persons with handicaps] are either oversexed and promiscuous, or have no sexual interest and should be regarded as children with a need to be protected from possible abuse. The former attitude reflects the view that we need to protect society from persons with handicaps; the latter view reflects the bias that we need to protect those individuals with handicaps from society. Both attitudes are equally restrictive and debilitating to the person with a developmental handicap ... This view also reflects a broader societal view of sexuality as negative and sinful" (p. 21). See also Coleman & Murphy (1980); Abramson, Parker, & Weisberg (1988).

[3] See Biklen & Mlinarcik (1978): "To date, extensive research—literally hundreds of studies—has revealed no unequivocal evidence to suggest a causal relationship between mental retardation and criminality. Yet popular culture, namely news accounts, still imply that the retarded are more prone to criminal acts or at least, that mental retardation is the cause of some criminal behavior" (p. 190).

[4] Although intellectually disabled females offend sexually—as do nondisabled females—males are presently in the preponderance of *identified* offenders in both populations. In a survey of 40 treatment providers reporting on 1567 intellectually disabled sex offenders (Knopp & Lackey, 1987), for example, all but 25 (1.6%) of the offenders were male. Intellectually disabled sex offenders are therefore referred to here as "he."

those posited by Lund, 1989) provide a multipurpose framework for looking at male sexuality:

1. Sexually relevant behavior and experiences are present across virtually all ages and developmental levels.
2. Adults experience great diversity in forms of sexual expression and preferences regardless of whether intellectual functioning is within or below "normal" limits.
3. These diverse forms of sexual expression reflect genetic, constitutional, physiological, developmental, and environmental influences, or may also reflect "accidents" of conditioning history, based on actual life experiences.
4. Sexual arousal and orgasm constitute a potent reinforcer; the pairing of heightened sexual arousal and orgasm with some object, event, fantasy, activity, or person produces powerful conditioned associations, attachments, and emotions.
5. Once this association occurs, it may promote the development of strong and unusual preferences.
6. Because sexual reinforcement is so powerful, it is difficult to alter preferences for certain types of sexual behavior except under the following conditions: (1) there is some acceptable alternative which is more reinforcing; (2) the specific sexual behavior produces negative consequences for the individual.

Despite commonalities in basic patterns of sexual behavior, there are marked differences in the historical and social context of the offending behavior of disabled and nondisabled sex offenders; issues of consent and competency[5] further complicate the situation. Nevertheless, the sexually aggressive behavior of intellectually disabled persons, like that of all sex offenders, must not be denied, minimized, or neglected. "Just as there is nothing inherent in the disability that makes men sex offenders," says Charlene Senn (1987) of the Roeher Institute of Toronto, Canada, "there is nothing inherent in it which would inoculate them from becoming one" (p. 90).

Offenses committed by intellectually disabled sex offenders generally parallel those of nondisabled offenders (Knopp & Lackey, 1987, pp. 5, 13-14; Safer Society Program, 1988, p. 4), though their "M.O.s" may

---

[5] For a discussion of informed and voluntary consent, see Griffiths, Quinsey, & Hingsburger (1989) pp. 173-182. See also Sgroi (1989) pp. 247-252.

differ. However, inappropriate or aggressive sexual behavior by intellectually disabled persons produces, with few exceptions, society's most negative responses, ranging from minimizing or ignoring these behaviors, to "revolving door" jail sentences, to harsh "warehousing" in maximum security institutions.[6] Whether disabled or nondisabled, the sex offender should be held responsible for his behavior and be provided access to a continuum of specialized remedial interventions.

Assessing & Treating Intellectually Disabled Sex Offenders

Based on clinical experience, many specialized treatment providers agree that intellectually disabled sex offenders, particularly those identified as in the "borderline" intellectually functioning range,[7] are surprisingly amenable to treatment (Fried, 1986, p. 2; Gafgen, 1988; Safer Society Program, 1988, p. 5). They are "cautiously optimistic" that with early recognition and intervention, the majority of ***low risk*** intellectually disabled sex offenders could benefit from treatment in specialized, individualized programs in the community (Griffiths, et al., p. 8). ***Moderate to higher risk*** offenders, on the other hand, require longer term, highly structured, creative programming in residential settings. Many clients in these higher risk categories have been treated with encouraging success in the residential Social Skills Program (see chapter 7).

Risk Issues

With all sex offenders, community safety is the primary issue in their assessment and treatment. This issue is not diminished for people with disabilities, although it may be complicated by the efforts of disability-rights advocates seeking to safeguard their constituents from overly intrusive treatment or potentially unwarranted intervention or incarceration. Moreover, intellectually disabled adult sex offenders' histories characteristically include early sexual victimization[8] in addition to other types of trauma and institutional and societal oppression. While such tragic and prejudicial

---

[6] Intellectually disabled offenders are overrepresented in prison populations, are usually imprisoned for longer periods of time, and have less access to alternative sentencing arrangements than nondisabled offenders. See Santamour (1986), pp. 7-10 for social and legal factors associated with their incarceration.

[7] IQs alone are not an adequate measure of an individual's cognitive or social abilities. In addition to cognitive deficits (indicated by IQ scores in the 55-84 range on the Wechsler Adult Intelligence Scale—Revised), these clients usually have serious adaptive skill deficits; they are typically represented in the Social Skills Program described in this book.

[8] In one study (Knopp & Lackey, 1987), treatment providers reported that 95% of the female and 68% of the male intellectually disabled sexual abusers related being sexually abused prior to offending (p. 4); Griffiths reports 100% of the offenders with developmental disabilities in her program as of June 1987 had been sexually abused as children (Senn, 1987, p. 102); Seattle Rape Relief (Crossmaker, 1986) estimates only 20% of sexual assaults perpetrated against people with intellectual disabilities are reported since 99% of their offenders are relatives, friends, acquaintances, or caretakers of the victim (p. 10).

experiences rightly evoke professional concern and sympathy, they should not prompt caring professionals to minimize or blur the risk factors involved in the client's sexually offending behavior. If the offender is at high risk to reoffend, such good but uninformed intentions are not helpful to the client or to the community.[9]

Although no validated offender typologies or longitudinal outcome studies based on specific models of treatment for adult sex offenders currently exist, working guidelines and data sources[10] used to assess risk for nondisabled sex offenders[11] are generally useful for assessing disabled clients. Some risk issues to be considered differentially in assessing intellectually disabled sex offenders[12] include:

• *Impulsivity.* Because internal controls may be lacking, the intellectually disabled sex offender's life may be characterized by an even greater degree of impulsivity than the nondisabled offender's. He generally is less able to project his life into the future and to understand the consequences of his actions. He may have a highly externalized "locus of control," perceiving many of the controlling factors in life as being "out there." As a result, he may feel frustrated and disempowered, unable to control what is happening to him (if he has been in residential care, this perception may have been fostered by those very institutions). He may be quick to anger, and, lacking verbal and social skills, have fewer ways to cope with his environment or divert his anger through cathartic release. A high degree of impulsive behavior in the client's nonsexual history may heighten his risk of offending sexually.

---

[9] Treatment staff at the Princeton, New Jersey, Moderate Security Counseling and Treatment Unit, for example, have been dealing with constant pressure to release clients to an environment of lesser restrictions. According to Senior Clinical Psychologist Eleanor R. Fried (1986): "Our dilemma is grave. While we are mandated by the courts to contain and treat dangerous sex offenders, we are also enjoined by the public advocate's office to engage in six-month retention hearings, where the burden of proof falls upon us to convince a hearing officer that these patients must remain for the welfare of society and themselves. The advocacy system today is such that should we not be able to prove our case, a sex offender may well be released before his treatment is completed ... Fortunately, I am here to tell you that we are inevitably successful in proving the case for treatment retention and the safety of society" (p. 6-7).

[10] In addition to evaluating data from indepth clinical interviews, client data are collected from social/sexual histories; self-reports; client journals and records; collateral information from law enforcement, court, institutional, and victim reports; psychophysiological and polygraph tests; and various other tests and measurements (Knopp & Lackey, 1987, p. 9). Practitioners view psychological, educational, and attitudinal tests as useful but not necessarily definitive. "If there is a contradiction between test results and the client's observed behavior, the behavior should be considered paramount in making the assessment" (Safer Society Program, 1989, p. 7).

[11] See Hall, 1989, pp. 48-68; Knopp, 1984, pp. 29-33; and Salter, 1988, pp. 182-205.

[12] Safer Society Program, 1988, pp. 4-5.

• *Predatory Behavior.* Intellectually disabled sex offenders appear to be less *covertly* predatory than nondisabled sex offenders. As previously mentioned, intellectually disabled sex offenders commit offenses that do not differ substantially from those committed by nondisabled sex offenders, except that they seldom establish consistent relationships with their victims. While the offenses of some may exhibit sophisticated victim-grooming patterns, they rarely involve specific age, gender, or appearance targets. In some cases, they may "grab" a more vulnerable victim on impulse and/or may not discriminate in their victims. Consequently, it may be more difficult to predict which "high risk" situations or specific age or gender group might trigger this type of offender's sexually aggressive behavior, placing him at higher risk for reoffending.

• *Use of Physical Force or Weapons.* As in all risk assessments, it is important to evaluate the type and degree of violence used in the commission of the sexual assault. Factors to be considered include whether the violence was *expressive* or *instrumental.* Those using *expressive* violence in the commission of the crime exhibit the highest risk for reoffending because the violence is intentional: the injury inflicted may be part of the offender's arousal pattern, not a means to ensure compliance. *Instrumental* violence, on the other hand, is characteristic of offenders who have lost control and use violence or the threat of violence to ensure compliance; use of violence, however, was not the original intent. The intellectually disabled sex offender is more likely to use instrumental violence, in part because he may lack the verbal skills of coaxing, bribing, and manipulating, and in part because of his low tolerance for frustration and tendency to panic in new situations.

• *Chronic Substance Abuse.* Chronic substance abuse exacerbates the lack of control and will-power characteristic of many intellectually disabled offenders, placing them at high risk for reoffending. (Few specialized treatment programs address these problems as comprehensively as the Social Skills Program's alcohol/drug treatment-focus area described in chapter 5.)

• *Firesetting, Animal Torture, and Enuresis.* The propensity for acting out aggressively appears to increase dramatically with intellectually disabled sex offenders whose histories contain a combination of firesetting, animal torture, and enuresis (bedwetting).[13] Setting fires to *occupied* dwellings places the intellectually disabled sex offender at higher risk to reoffend.

---

[13] All three elements must be present to correlate with increased risk. Enuresis is uncommon among nondisabled adult sex offenders.

• *Failed Prior Specialized Treatment.* This risk criterion should be used with extreme caution in evaluating intellectually disabled sex offenders. While any client who reoffends *during or after completing* a specialized sex-offender treatment program is considered higher risk, with intellectually disabled sex offenders, the *quality* of previous treatment should first be carefully explored before making this assessment. Prior treatment may have been inappropriate to the client's needs, or he may have been main-streamed in an institutional setting without appropriate support. In such cases, rather than automatically moving the client to a secure residential setting, probation with more restrictive and intrusive monitoring and intensive community programming may suffice.

Treatment Settings and Options

Recent surveys (Knopp & Stevenson, 1989) indicate that 43% of the identified specialized sex-offender treatment programs in the United States provide some sort of services for intellectually disabled clients,[14] but they are rarely adequate or comprehensive. The majority of programs provide weekly individual one-hour counseling sessions and/or integrate the disabled client into groups with nondisabled sex offenders, slowing down and repeating sex-offender-specific treatment procedures in more concrete form. There are relatively few comprehensive community-based or residential programs available to intellectually disabled sex offenders, though the need is compelling.[15]

Sex-offender treatment professionals and advocates for the disabled both prefer the least restrictive settings and interventions possible while ensuring community and client safety. But such placements are only possible when a continuum of specialized treatment and care in a variety of living environments is available: community outpatient, supported living arrangements in the community, day school, and open or closed residential settings. With a full range of treatment options, clients can move to different levels of independence as indicated by their behavior and treatment needs. The innovative Social Skills Program described in this book represents one

---

[14] Some type of specialized treatment for intellectually disabled clients was indicated by 43% (183) of all 429 identified *adult* specialized sex-offender service providers and 43% (247) of all 573 *juvenile* service providers surveyed by The Safer Society Program. Services are unevenly distributed geographically: 25% of adult services for the intellectually disabled sex offender population are located in four states (California, Illinois, Minnesota, and Washington), and five states (California, Massachusetts, Ohio, Oregon, and Washington) host 39% of juvenile services to this population (Knopp & Stevenson, 1989, p. 19).

[15] More than half of all requests for sex-offender assessment and treatment referrals received in 1989 by The Safer Society Program's National Referral Service are related to intellectually disabled clients. Only a limited number of such requests can be accommodated because of lack of specialized services.

important and rare part of that continuum—an intensive residential treatment model in a closed setting with a variety of specialized aftercare arrangements in supervised dorms, sheltered housing, and community placements.

Treatment Needs

While experienced clinicians who work with both disabled and nondisabled sex offenders recognize more similarities than differences between the two populations, there is an appalling lack of research, studies, and treatment models in the literature to assist in treatment planning for intellectually disabled sex offenders compared to the treatment resources available for nondisabled sex offenders (Murphy, Coleman, & Haynes, 1983, pp. 22-23). This lack of resources for intellectually disabled sex offenders can be remedied when clinicians treating sex offenders and professionals (especially sex educators) working with intellectually disabled populations combine their skills and experience. By merging their expertise and knowledge, these professionals will be better able to identify the most effective treatment components and teaching modalities for intellectually disabled sex offenders. *Treating Intellectually Disabled Sex Offenders: A Model Residential Program* is intended to assist that process by describing the unique Social Skills Program housed in the Oregon State Hospital.

Part I provides the framework for an indepth understanding of the treatment components described in Part II. Chapter 1 reviews how the Social Skills Program (SSP) came into being; provides a basic description of its services and physical setting; outlines staff responsibilities and training; and delineates the population the program serves as well as its entrance criteria. Chapter 2 defines the SSP's unique treatment milieu, incorporating a *modified* therapeutic community, individualized treatment planning, and the concrete application of self-help principles. Chapter 3 discusses similarities and differences in treating intellectually disabled and nondisabled sex offenders with regard to selected clinical issues and methodologies.

Part II presents the treatment components of the SSP. It begins with the case study of Kevin, illustrating the background and Orientation treatment for a "typical" client. Chapter 4 provides a detailed description of the SSP's Orientation phase, including assessment, support and treatment groups, and basic workshops. Preceded by the case study of Kevin's Inhouse treatment, chapter 5 describes the Inhouse treatment phase: general treatment approaches; five treatment-focus areas, including a discussion of personality disorder as related to intellectually disabled sex offenders; specific adaptations of cognitive/behavioral interventions; and examples of projects used to teach social skill concepts. The case study of Kevin's Transition treatment precedes chapter 6, which details the SSP's Transition treatment phase and Pre-release/Aftercare program to help the client develop skills, strategies, and support for offense-free living in the community. Following chapter 6, Steve is introduced in a detailed case study illustrating the eclectic and prescriptive qualities of the SSP's approach to holistic treatment. Chapter 7 reviews available outcome data, along with some less quantifiable benefits of treatment for the offender, the community, and treatment and corrections agencies.

The SSP is constantly evolving in creative ways; this manual describes the program as of November 1989. It is written from a "systems" point of view, so that other programs using this model can discover their own specific adaptations and teaching methods to fill in the detailed substance. Such freedom helps staff and clients to express their creativity and "own" their process, both basic principles of the SSP.

Finally, as publishers, we celebrate the skills and creativity of the dedicated professionals at the SSP who are working steadfastly with clients whom society would prefer to ignore, punish, or shut away forever. We applaud their willingness to try over and over again with difficult clients and their reluctance to give up and permanently expel clients from the program when they appear to fail. In practice, they are reaffirming the essential humanity of the intellectually disabled sex offender by insisting that he take responsibility for his acts and by providing him with hope and the possibility that he may learn an acceptable lifestyle. Such efforts are compelling and worthy of our support; they will rnake our communities more humane and safer from sexual assault.

Fay Honey Knopp
The Safer Society Program and Press
Orwell, Vermont
January, 1990

1

PROGRAM HISTORY AND DESCRIPTION

Oregon State Hospital's Social Skills Program (SSP) is designed for intellectually disabled offenders who display habitual patterns of criminal behavior and would usually be sentenced to prison with little likelihood of corrective treatment. Sex offenders now comprise 90% of the SSP's population and have been receiving specialized treatment since 1983. This manual describes in detail the residential social skills treatment and transition program.

History

Since 1975 Oregon's Department of Corrections and Department of Human Resources' Mental Health and Developmentally Disabled Division have joined cooperatively in developing, operating, and maintaining mental health services for Department of Corrections clients. In November 1978 the administrators of those agencies entered into a cooperative agreement spelling out specific responsibilities for providing services to clients under the jurisdiction of the Department of Corrections. This cooperative agreement established the ground rules under which the Correctional Treatment Programs (CTP)[1] currently operate.

Because of the unique cooperative nature of the CTP, the legislature in 1975 established the Mental Health Programs under oversight of the Corrections Policy Board.[2] It establishes broad policies governing the operation of the Mental Health Programs in Corrections, including the administrative rules of transfer.[3] The first clients were transferred from their parent institutions to the Mentally/Emotionally Disturbed Program, the Sex Offender Program, and the SSP in September 1979.

---

[1] Five distinct programs provide treatment services for clients in Oregon Department of Corrections facilities under the umbrella of the CTP: the Cornerstone Alcohol and Drug Treatment Program, the Mentally/Emotionally Disturbed Program, the Sex Offender Program, the Correctional Institution Treatment Services (a consultant program for prison residents), and the SSP.

[2] The Policy Board includes the assistant administrators of both divisions, institutional superintendents from the state community mental health programs directors' association, and the director of the CTP.

[3] These rules set forth terms and conditions under which a client is transferred from his or her parent institution to the CTP at the Oregon State Hospital.

Program Description

The SSP is a unique treatment alternative for adjudicated intellectually disabled offenders with limited adaptive skills who need both intensive treatment and a controlled safe environment. The program provides:

- long-term intensive programming combining the latest technology with modalities adapted to the client's disabilities;
- comprehensive treatment—including a strong chemical dependency treatment module—occurring 24 hours a day in a secure setting separate from the prison's "con" culture;
- training in self-help that counters institutional dependence;
- treatment methodologies that engage the client's emotions as well as addressing his behaviors and thoughts;
- a supportive, firm, spontaneous, and consistent treatment atmosphere;
- extensive transition services with community follow-up;
- education, training, and networking of resources and methods for the wider community.

Treatment takes place in three stages: *Orientation*, lasting 60-90 days (see chapter 4); *Inhouse treatment*, lasting 9-36 months (see chapter 5);[4] and *Transition treatment*, lasting 6-9 months (see chapter 6).[5] Thereafter, supervision continues while the client is on parole: one of the conditions of parole is the continuing supervision of treatment by the SSP for 12-24 months, providing a consistency of treatment that enhances the chances of successful community transition.

Physical Setting

The SSP is located in a 31-bed secure unit on the third floor of the original state hospital, a building characteristic of late nineteenth century architecture. Similar in layout to a hospital psychiatric ward, the unit consists of a long hall with side rooms for treatment activities and living areas. Three to four residents share small dorm sleeping areas; each resident has his own unlocked bedroom. The program has access to a dining

---

[4] SSP staff do not concentrate on long-term treatment since approximately half of the program's clients leave within nine months. Because many offenders do not complete treatment, modules are short-term; success is then possible for clients who complete their treatment in just one or two of the five possible treatment areas.

[5] This phase is similar to prison "work-release": clients work outside the institution while living on the unit.

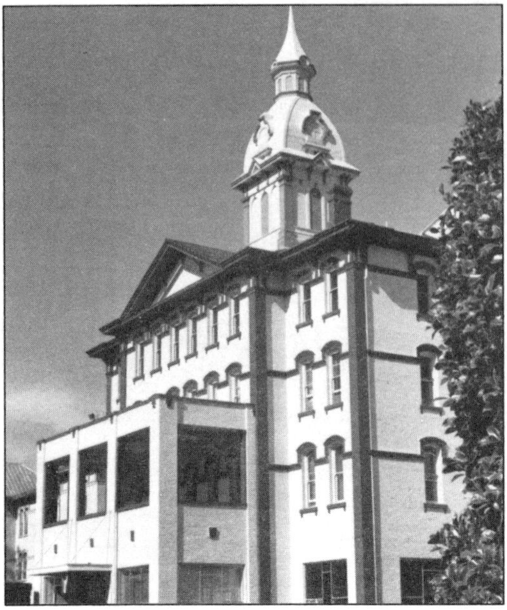

Oregon State Hospital, Salem, OR

room, chapel area, music room, cooking facilities, and a gymnasium with side rooms for ceramics, as well as a fenced-in yard area outside. All activities areas are within a fenced security perimeter monitored by TV cameras; residents can leave the secure perimeter only when they are in the community transition phase of treatment.

Staff

The SSP has two organizational systems: one details program operational duties (outreach, security, resident escort, and other facility upkeep responsibilities) and is supervised by Correctional Treatment Therapists (CTTs); the second system outlines the clinical structure of the SSP (see Appendix A).

Twenty-one full-time and three part-time staff[6] direct the SSP. The staff Psychiatrist, Psychologist, and Educational Specialist report to the CTP Director and are accountable to the SSP Director. Interns and graduate students serve as adjunctive staff. Student interns in art and music therapy, therapeutic recreation, education, psychology, nursing, and health rec-

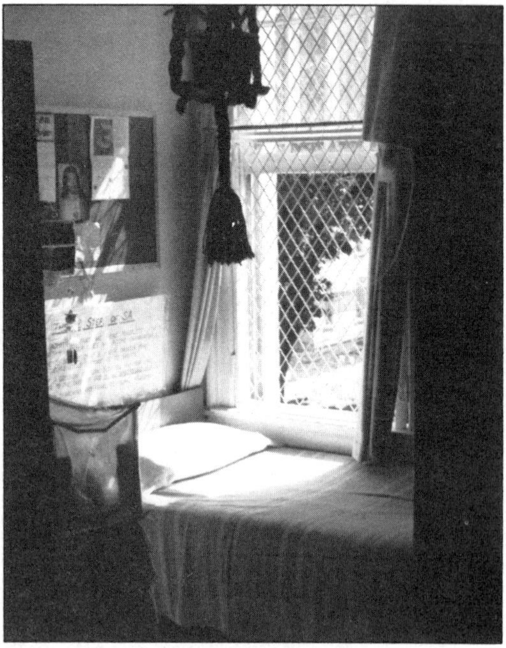

A resident's bedroom

[6] Full-time staff consist of the Director, 2 Inhouse Therapy Supervisors, 1 Aftercare Therapy Supervisor, 1 Recreational Therapist, 1 Registered Nurse, and 15 CTTs. Part-time staff include a 1/3-time Psychiatrist, 1/3-time Psychologist, and a 3/4-time Educational Specialist.

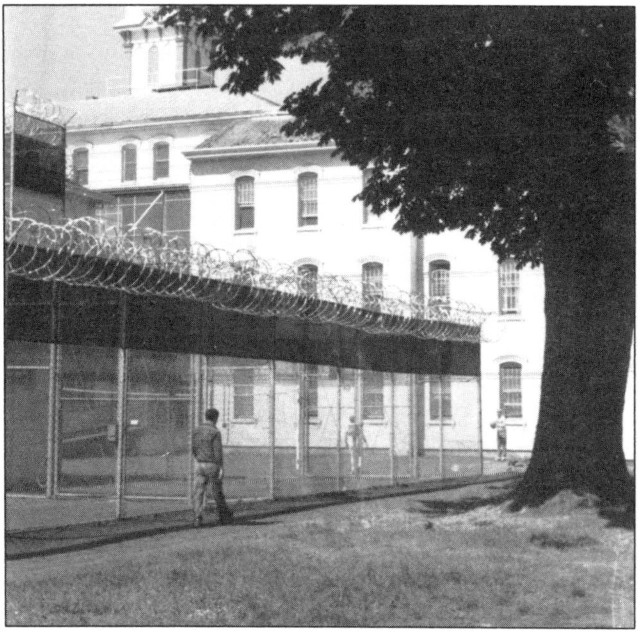

TV-monitored security perimeter

ords-keeping work with the SSP along with graduate students in counseling, social work, and theology. Interns and students are clinically supervised by one of the three Therapy Supervisors and meet monthly with the Director. Eventually they may conduct groups or workshops in their disciplines and fully participate as staff members.

Believing that the program is only as creative, productive, and effective as its staff, administrators encourage them to develop a clear sense of territory and ownership of specific points of programming and give recognition for their efforts. Work schedules allow time for creative expression and quality performance. The work environment is team-oriented and supportive; respect and humor are valued. Because of their clients' multiple diagnoses, staff have developed a broad range of expertise. While individual staff specialize in various treatment modalities and retain responsibility for overseeing modules within their special expertise, they periodically rotate assignments to broaden their understanding of all the treatment components and to promote integration.

Staff Training

The program's organizational design and its quest for quality treatment foster staff growth through comprehensive training and ongoing clinical supervision. The Oregon State Hospital requires 40 hours of training for all new staff, including instruction in how to manage aggressive behavior. Permanent, full-time staff are required to have an additional eight hours of training yearly. CTTs working in the behavioral laboratory[7] must complete an intensive 28-hour classroom training program and provide 60 hours of direct treatment under close supervision. They learn and use diagnostic terminology as a common language for sharing information with each other and with other professionals.

Staff members are encouraged to attend workshops and seminars, to read new literature in research and treatment, and to seek training in topics relevant to the SSP (neuro-psychology, anger management, use of the *DSM III-R*,[8] counseling techniques, workshop presentation techniques, sex-offender treatment, and so forth). The Alcohol and Drug Program Office of the Mental Health Division provides week-long training in the assessment and treatment of alcohol and drug problems. Additional training opportunities for staff are available through the SSP's contacts with other agencies in the community and through co-worker inservice training sessions.

Semiannually, all SSP staff members participate in a retreat where they receive intensive training, discuss major program changes or additions, address staff issues or concerns, and build cohesiveness and morale.

Population Served

Residents in the SSP may have serious psychiatric and/or neurological problems, sexual deviancy, and/or character disorders. All share the common problem of being designated as intellectually disabled, falling into the mild mental retardation (IQ range 55-69: 20% of the SSP population) and borderline intellectually functioning ranges (IQ range 70-85: 80% of the SSP population).[9] Approximately 25 percent of the residents have Axis I diagnoses[10] of mental illness; 85 percent have serious alcohol or poly-drug-

---

[7] The behavioral laboratory is the setting for conducting sexual arousal assessments and deviant arousal reduction training. See chapter 5 for more detailed information.

[8] The *Diagnostic and Statistical Manual of Mental Disorders Third Edition—Revised* (American Psychiatric Association, 1987) is a compilation of accepted diagnoses used by researchers, clinicians, and insurance companies for classification purposes.

[9] Traditionally, because they do not fit the American Association for Mental Deficiencies classification for the mentally retarded, persons in the borderline intellectually functioning range rarely are provided special services.

[10] The *DSM III-R* (American Psychiatric Association, 1987) establishes five categories or "axes" to aid clinicians and researchers in evaluating and classifying mental disorders. Axis I covers "clinical syndromes" and "conditions not attributable to a mental disorder that are a focus of attention or treatment." Axis II includes "developmental disorders and personality disorders ... [which] generally begin in childhood or adolescence and persist in stable form ... into adult life." Axis III represents "physical disorders or conditions ... potentially relevant to the understanding or management of the case" (pp. 16, 18). See the *DSM III-R* for a detailed explanation of these categories.

abuse problems, and almost all have character disorders. It is common to have a client who is developmentally disabled, mentally or emotionally disturbed, sexually deviant, alcoholic, and severely personality-disordered with an entrenched criminal value system. On average, their reading/math skills are on a fourth- to fifth-grade level. Over 70 percent of the residents show signs of organicity.[11]

Organicity

Of 31 SSP clients, 23 (74%) had been diagnosed as having an organic mental syndrome.[12] Of these 23 residents, 20 were convicted sex offenders, and three committed sexually related crimes (such as assaulting lovers over nonsexual matters). While organicity has played a major or minor role in the offenses of each of these 20 intellectually disabled sex offenders, this apparent relationship should not be generalized to the organically impaired intellectually disabled population as a whole. The most commonly described change in sexual behavior related to organic brain damage cited in the literature has been that of *decreased* libido; however, sexual disinhibition, hypersexuality, and change in sexual preference have also been reported (Blumer, 1970; Koloday, Masters, & Johnson, 1979, p. 254; Miller, Cummings, McIntyre, Ebers, & Grode, 1986; Weinstein, 1974). Common additional effects of organicity include poor abstract reasoning, inability to sequence events, little memory recall, aggressive behaviors, explosiveness, and anxiety disorders.

The percentage of brain-injured intellectually disabled offenders in the SSP (74%) appears startling until compared with the percentage of *nondisabled* offenders who are brain injured. One study of 160 incarcerated sex offenders, for example, demonstrated a rate of organicity as high as 50 percent (Graber, Hartman, Coffman, Huey, & Goldy, 1982). Nevertheless, SSP residents appear to be more impaired than nondisabled brain-injured offenders because they have additional learning disabilities exacerbated by their organicity.[13]

While there are no known cures for organic mental syndromes, some treatment interventions can be tailored to lessen their effect. The SSP integrates allowances for organic difficulties into each group, counseling

---

[11] Organicity is a psychological or behavioral abnormality associated with transient or permanent dysfunction of the brain. The dysfunction may be genetic or trauma-induced.

[12] Historically this proportion has ranged from 50 percent to 75 percent of the unit population. These figures relate to the SSP as of November 1989.

[13] While residents lack adaptive skills, they seem to have greater "street survival" skills than is traditional for institutionalized persons with intellectual deficits.

session, activity, class, and workshop. Examples of program adaptations are included throughout this manual.

Multiple Diagnoses

Because of organicity, affective disorders, mental retardation, sexual deviancy, or alcohol/drug abuse, intellectually disabled offenders may have a wider and more complex constellation of problems. For example, Ralph, an organically impaired client, had poor coping skills, low self-esteem, and disabling emotional disorders. He was incarcerated for molesting a three-year-old neighbor girl. In addition to pedophilia, he was diagnosed as having a generalized anxiety disorder, alcohol dependence, and an avoidant personality disorder.

It is not the severity of any single diagnosis that makes treatment difficult but rather the combination and interplay of multiple problems. An individual may be an alcoholic, have schizophrenic symptoms, moderate organic brain impairment, and an IQ of 73 and still not qualify for any state-funded institutional or community services. While none of these conditions by itself may be severe enough to qualify for state-provided services, the cumulative effect is severely disabling. Even when services are offered, their programming usually addresses a higher-functioning client, making it difficult or impossible for an intellectually disabled individual to benefit.

Offender Typologies

The 27 convicted sex offenders in the SSP in November 1989 could be divided into five typologies by offense dynamic. Of the 23 pedophiles, 9 were regressed; 6 were fixated; and 8 were pansexual offenders. Of the 4 rapists with adult victims, 2 were sadistic and 2 were frustration/anger rapists.

The nine regressed pedophiles preferred adult partners but committed sexual offenses against children under specific circumstances. When assessed, they demonstrated some arousal to children, but appeared to act out that interest only under highly stressful situations such as divorce, loss of job, health problems, and heavy drinking.

The offenses of the six fixated pedophiles showed elements of obsession and compulsion. These six men had well defined sexual preferences not only in the gender of their victims, but also in a specific narrow age range. They were often additionally fixated on such factors as color of hair, complexion, body type, clothing, or vulnerable looks. They reported that they felt psychological discomfort when a target matching their preferred image was not accessible. Their offenses involved alcohol and stress factors less often than those of the regressed offenders. Male children were their most frequent targets.

The eight pansexual pedophiles often verbalized same-sex preferences, but in reality they were opportunistic. Regardless of sex or age, any available partner, willing or unwilling, was acceptable. They had a high frequency of acting out.

The primary sexual interest of the two sadistic rapists was inflicting pain and suffering on their victims. One was opportunistic and committed three rapes: two against females and one against a male. The other had many victims in carefully plotted circumstances. Both had histories of family violence and abandonment, and both had been institutionalized at an early age.

The two frustration/anger rapists raped after being rejected by their victims. Both experienced organically based hallucinations and had borderline personality features. Both exhibited bipolar symptoms which partially responded to lithium carbonate.

Entrance Criteria

To be considered for entrance into the SSP, potential participants must be incarcerated in one of the state's four adult correctional institutions and have one to four years of their sentences remaining. Clients may make application directly to the SSP or may be referred by their institutional counselors or teachers, family members, courts, or others. Because the SSP is voluntary, clients cannot be transferred without their approval.

The SSP Director interviews the prospective client while he is still in his correctional institution. There are three criteria for acceptance into the program: (1) the client must express willingness to come into the program; (2) he must be designated in the borderline intellectual functioning range or lower with serious adaptive skill deficits (IQ range 55-84 on the WAIS-R[14]); and (3) the client must be *amenable* to treatment, that is, the defenses that support his "old" offending identity can be fragmented within six months of admission or he can be convinced that this program offers his last, best hope for staying out of prison in the future, indicating a reasonable prognosis for change to a "new" nonoffending identity.

Once the client has been accepted for treatment, notification of acceptance is mailed to his correctional institution. The institution sends to

---

[14] Wechsler Adult Intelligence Scale—Revised; see Resources.

the SSP a complete packet of information, including the client's offense history, presentence investigation report, and institutional record. He is placed on the waiting list until a bed becomes available and is then transported to the SSP.

TREATMENT MILIEU AND APPROACHES

Recognizing that a global change must take place in the client's values, behaviors, and perceptions, SSP treatment approaches are comprehensive and eclectic. A multidisciplinary Treatment Team coordinates the multidiagnostic approach to a wide range of client disorders and disabilities.[1] The modified therapeutic community, incorporating individualized treatment planning, is the primary agent of change.

The Treatment Milieu

The SSP's *modified therapeutic community*[2] is based on two premises: all behavior within the program environment is relevant to treatment; and the resident is capable of taking a responsible role in the functioning of the unit and in understanding his own behavior (self-help). Staff's role is to assist the resident to act, initiate, cooperate, and manage his own affairs. Staff and residents view any deviation from responsibility as an opportunity to refocus the resident's attention on his behavior and its effects on other people. Therefore, immediate treatment intervention occurs at the time of the irresponsible behavior.

The SSP milieu includes a warm, respectful, humane, and consistent environment and the development of a communal feeling between residents and staff. The program is dynamic, creating an atmosphere of tasks still to be done or changed—a sense of ragged edges and unfinished business—

---

[1] The Treatment Team is made up of the SSP's Director, Psychiatrist, Psychologist, Therapy Supervisors, Educational Specialist, Recreational Therapist, Registered Nurse, and Correctional Treatment Therapist (CTT).

[2] The trademark of the pure therapeutic community model, as defined by Jones (1953), is the community meeting where all staff and residents address community problems. Full community meetings do not occur in the SSP because they create an unrealistic forum for problem solving compared to what clients will find in the noninstitutional community. More importantly, with offender populations the community meeting usually reinforces rather than treats their pathological issues, providing a grand stage (complete with audience) on which to act out. The SSP has found that increased involvement, ability to compromise, and patience is fostered by directing residents to work out issues in small groups and then coordinating their solutions to meet the needs of the entire community. Also, pure therapeutic communities focus on the client's making an intense commitment to the community, merging his identity into that of the community. The SSP encourages the development of a singular identity in each of its clients through the use of individualized treatment plans and graded responsibilities. Further, pure therapeutic communities often rely on cathartic confession rituals to create movement; the SSP does not.

within a defined structure (see Appendix B for Treatment Schedule). Essentially, the community is designed as an effective educational process where residents feel they can take risks. All aspects of the program are considered potential opportunities for skill building, increasing knowledge, and clarifying values. The focus is on challenge without failure, and the learning environment is relaxed and supportive. Reinforcement is generated by the residents themselves, while workshop trainers provide structure and act as facilitators.

Four principles define the SSP's modified therapeutic community:

• *Every task that can be organized and performed by residents is allocated to them.* In traditional institutional programs, staff act as caregivers, assuming many daily operational, educational, and clinical responsibilities rather than encouraging the residents to decide how to handle these responsibilities themselves. In the SSP, however, a resident with a question or concern is encouraged to take it to one of his peers first. When resolution is not possible at that level, he goes to a staff person for assistance. "Buddy" arrangements allow residents to help each other and foster a cooperative relationship that relies less on staff assistance.

• *The process is more important than the task being performed.* Treatment focuses on reasoning and problem solving in daily issues and tasks rather than on the final result. The resident learns by trying new things, making mistakes, taking risks, working with others, and learning through trial and error. Though staff tend to focus on task completion, the residents generalize information and understanding through trial and error in a forum where interventions into their pathologies can take place. For example, in a gardening class, a productive garden is not the primary measure of success; the primary focus is on creating a learning and treatment experience where people work together and develop an understanding of themselves and others.

• *Demonstration creates more change than telling the resident "how."* Experiential and application learning, using role playing, are more effective than didactic instruction and insight discussion. Such demonstrations occur in mini-role plays by residents and staff when differences arise on the unit. Staff and residents discuss possible choices and their consequences, rather than verbally confronting the participants.

• *An open communication system allows staff and residents to express thoughts and feelings honestly.* Open and direct communication is essential in a modified therapeutic community, providing an atmosphere that fosters dignity and self-respect. Creating multiple channels of communication

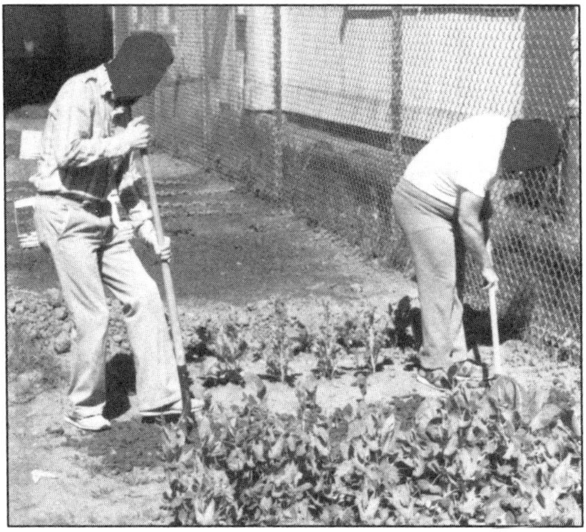

Learning to work together in the garden

within the treatment community enables residents to share their concerns and issues in responsible ways and in a comfortable manner. Communication channels include discussions in treatment groups, individual meetings with peers, individual counseling with staff, and daily journals. Expressive therapies, such as music and art, help residents communicate issues and feelings that are normally threatening for them to share.

All communication on the unit is unconditionally respectful; residents and staff refrain from threats, profanity, or street jargon. High level confrontation or "attack therapy" is prohibited. The resident must feel that he will be helped, motivated, and encouraged to achieve his maximum potential; responsibilities are clearly outlined; and he knows where to go, to whom, and for what, opening the way for independent learning.

Treatment Approaches

Using individualized treatment planning, SSP programming focuses on creating a total change in how each client relates to himself and the world. The resident is placed in a position where his old ways of thinking and behaving do not meet his basic survival needs within the modified therapeutic community. Working through an "old me—new me" identification process, the resident learns how to establish his new identity, fragmenting and discarding each piece of his old identity over time. Treatment approaches used in effecting this change include:

- *Re-parenting.* Through a process of moral development the resident learns how to identify values with behaviors. Staff and peers reinforce behaviors demonstrating empathy, openness, and honesty.

• *Changing the offender's thinking as well as his behavior.* Traditionally, treatment programs include some type of technique to influence the offender's thinking (Knopp & Stevenson, 1989; Ross, Fabiano, & Earles, 1988). Often overlooked as a treatment technique for intellectually disabled offenders, cognitive restructuring is effective with this population if interventions are adapted to their individual learning problems and limited reasoning abilities. Residents learn through a simple labeling approach to recognize and change their thinking patterns. Insight training is de-emphasized.

• *Linking emotion to the learning process.* To enhance the resident's ability to retain what he has learned, programming emphasizes the affective element of the learning process, using play as an approach to teaching life and treatment skills. Residents retain what they are taught if the learning experience is fun, dramatic, or bizarre.

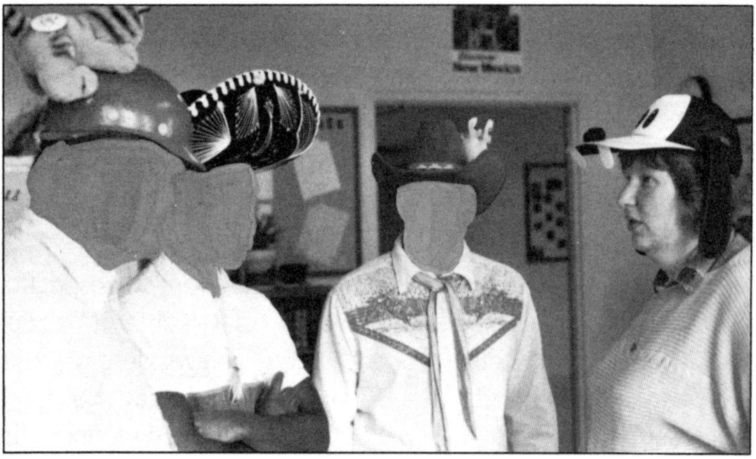

"Fun, dramatic, or bizarre": International Hat Day

• *Teaching keyed to the resident's multiple intelligences.* Since all people learn through at least seven intelligences (linguistic, logical/mathematical, intrapersonal, spatial, musical, bodily/kinesthetic, and interpersonal; Gardner, 1983), the SSP teaches concepts and skills using art, music, dance, role-playing, and other creative nontraditional activities.[3]

• *Using the group process.* Residents work in Orientation and Inpatient treatment groups, support groups, and later in a Pre-release/Aftercare group. These groups reinforce the behavioral and cognitive changes clients learn in workshops, classes, and other activities (see chapter 4). In the

[3] For example, staff might teach spelling through having the client spell words on a (waterproof) wall using a squirt gun.

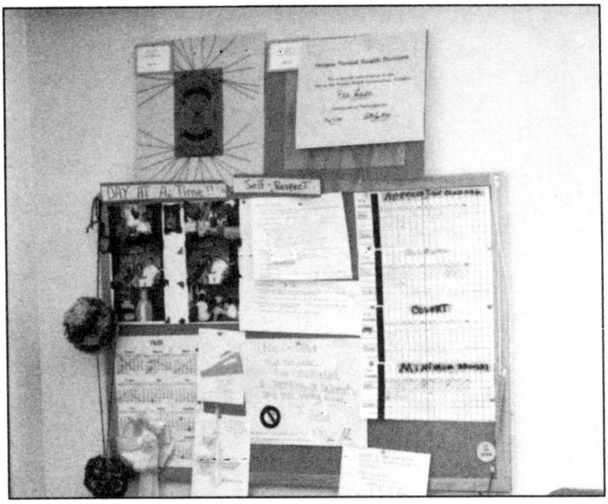

Bulletin board in a resident's room

program's group work (based on Santamour & West, 1979), SSP clients find they:

- — are treated with respect;
- — can express their ideas honestly;
- — can develop interpersonal skills in a safe place;
- — learn to deal with rules and authority figures;
- — can experiment with appropriate anger display;
- — can overcome self-imposed isolation and learn healthier ways of dealing with others;
- — learn impulse control;
- — observe staff participants modeling how to work with their issues.

• *Organizing the environment.* In residential treatment programs, the enthusiasm for using specific treatment techniques often overshadows the importance of the physical environment. In the SSP, the treatment environment is designed specifically to foster behavioral and cognitive change (Willis, 1980). Each resident has a private space, providing him with security for his possessions and permitting him to make his own choices about needing time to be by himself. Residents pin certificates, family pictures, and other items of interest on private bulletin boards. In order to personalize their sleeping areas, some residents make their own bedspreads and grow plants. Private space is also available on the unit, giving them a choice of spaces and allowing them time to be away from other residents.

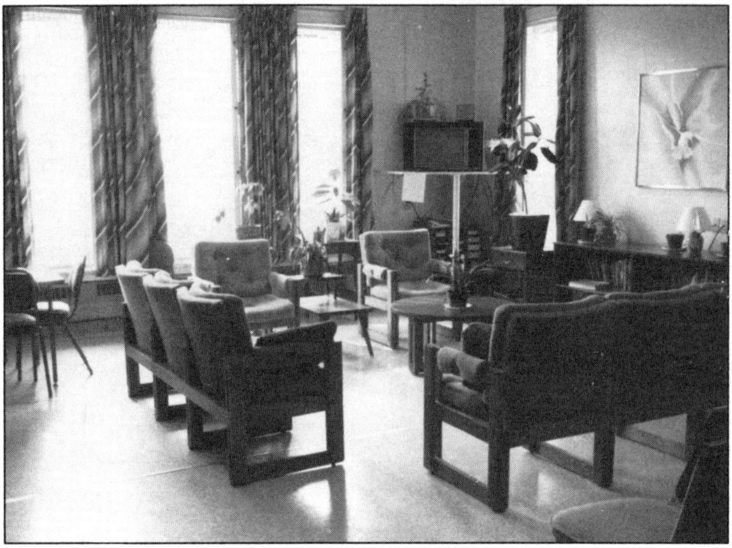

The dayroom

The day room, designed and furnished as a warm and comfortable home living room with floor lamps rather than overhead lighting, is the primary social space for all residents. Space planning provides defined areas allowing residents to read, watch television, or socialize. TV is allowed after 9:00 p.m. and on weekends.

Much of the unit's recreational activity is in group-room areas for meetings and workshops. Staff encourage residents to visit social areas during their free time. At small tables intended to promote socialization, they can find puzzles, art equipment, a stereo, an aquarium, and books. There is even a unit pet!

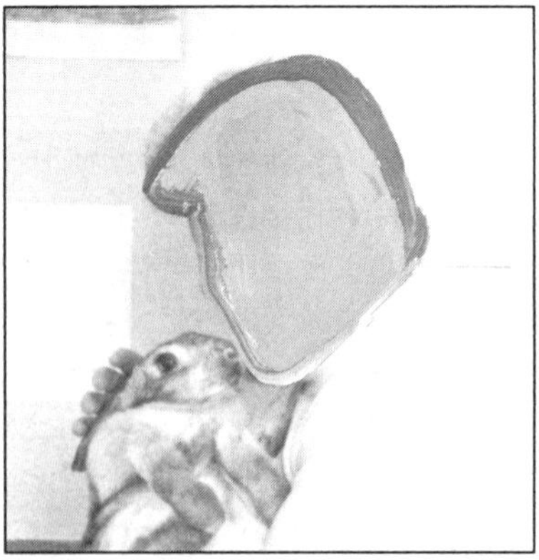

Gypsy, the unit pet

3

TREATING DISABLED AND NONDISABLED SEX OFFENDERS: SIMILARITIES AND DIFFERENCES

Treatment Issues

There are more similarities than differences in working with intellectually disabled sex offenders compared to nondisabled sex offenders. Characteristically, both groups have complex cognitive and behavioral deficits. They express various levels of denial; possess immature social and sexual skills, leading to helplessness and lack of assertiveness; feel intimidated by peers; experience low self-esteem and high self-criticism; demonstrate inadequate adult heterosexual or homosexual responsivity; engage in obsessively deviant fantasy patterns; lack empathy; display poor impulse control, particularly in response to stress; are unable to process and evaluate information, particularly about sexual roles and sexuality; and so forth (Schwartz & Masters, 1983).

Three primary issues exemplify similarities and differences between intellectually disabled and nondisabled sex offender populations: *denial, coping and learning skills,* and *self-esteem.* While they hardly comprise a comprehensive list, they represent problems experienced by sex offenders in general.

Denial

Disabled and nondisabled sex offenders are similar in their wide degree of variability in denial: some deny the offense completely while others quibble over the frequency and the amount of force used. Both groups have developed self-serving thought processes justifying their acts.

The "thinking errors"[1] involved in the denial by both groups show no significant difference in sophistication: the college graduate is as likely as the special education graduate to say, "I didn't think the six-year-old would remember." In both groups the most elaborate rationales are used by

[1] The term "thinking errors," called "criminal thinking" by Yochelson & Samenow (1976-77), describes distortions in thought and emotion used to justify "criminal" behavior. They include rationalization, polarized thinking, minimization, denial, anger, and lying, among others. These "thinking errors" are virtually always displayed by both disabled and nondisabled sex offenders.

offenders who employ subtle coercion as a means of getting victimized family members or acquaintances to cooperate in the abuse. Also, in both groups, offenders committing nonsituational crimes in more aggressive ways seem to have the least developed rationales.

Once in treatment, however, nondisabled and disabled sex offenders appear to respond differently when their denial is questioned. Many nondisabled offenders quickly appear to abandon their prior protestations of denial, often using such phrases as, "I woke up," or "It dawned on me what I was doing." However, this ready response can be quite superficial; in reality, they are extending their denial to their well-entrenched justification system, making effective treatment more difficult. Intellectually disabled offenders, on the other hand, tend to cling to their justification systems more rigidly. Progress is slow but more likely real.

A frontal attack on denial has not been effective with intellectually disabled offenders in the SSP; their denial is reduced using an incremental disclosure approach, supported by arousal assessment data and peer and staff tutors (for a detailed description, see the Sexual Deviancy Treatment-focus Area section in chapter 5).

Coping and Learning Skills

Intellectually disabled offenders have greater difficulty taking care of themselves and solving life crises than nondisabled offenders. They are more dependent on the program and staff, resulting in better compliance with program rules and a continuing association with the program long after they are free from any legal requirements.

Self-esteem

Self-esteem is a particularly difficult issue for intellectually disabled sex offenders. Both disabled and nondisabled sex offenders suffer from low self-esteem; however, the nondisabled offenders have a broader range of competencies allowing more positive social interactions. Because disabled offenders have fewer areas of competency, they compensate by exaggerating their accomplishments, a tendency others often see as abrasive and obnoxious. Also, they are sensitive to criticism; overreact to feedback from others; are more fearful of change because it is so difficult for them; and try to hang onto behaviors they have mastered, even when they are only minimally adaptive.

Treatment Methods

Since 1979, the SSP has pioneered innovative treatment methods.[2] By carefully discarding what did not work and retaining what did, the program has evolved into a unique collection of effective treatment components described in Part II of this manual. The section below identifies (1) cognitive/behavioral interventions that have proven effective contrary to expectations; (2) various interventions that have only limited application; and (3) interventions that have not been effective with this disabled sex-offender population.

Unexpectedly Effective Interventions

Because of the misconception that they are unable to change their thinking patterns, *cognitive restructuring* has seldom been used in the treatment of intellectually disabled sex offenders. However, with methods adapted to their particular learning problems, the SSP uses cognitive restructuring successfully with this population. Insight training, requiring the resident to use inductive and deductive reasoning skills, is de-emphasized. Instead, teaching is designed around a simple labeling approach. The resident is taught to associate a particular label with a constellation of behaviors or thoughts, enabling him to identify and associate new thoughts or behaviors with new labels (see chapter 5).

Minimal Arousal Conditioning and Covert Sensitization[3] have proven as effective and generalize as well for intellectually disabled offenders as they do for nondisabled offenders (Steinhauser, 1989). However, since gains deteriorate somewhat faster, maintenance sessions are more frequent, and longer follow-up periods are necessary.

Plethysmography[4] is used in the cognitive/behavioral interventions mentioned above. When adapted for intellectually disabled offenders, plethysmography is useful in a number of ways:

• *Treatment focuses on deviant arousal and behaviors.* Intellectually disabled sex offenders often have so many interrelated problems it is easy to lose sight of the specific aberrant behaviors that initially led them to the SSP. Plethysmography clarifies for staff the client's deviant behavioral patterns. After the assessment, treatment is tailored to the individual client's arousal and behavioral patterns.

• *A valid psychophysiological evaluation helps clients lessen their denial.* A review of direct behavioral evidence with a client often leads to the

---

[2] See Knopp (1984), pp. 202-209 for a description of the SSP after five years of program development.

[3] See chapter 5 for an explanation of these techniques as adapted by the SSP.

[4] *Plethysmography* (also referred to as penile plethysmography and psychophysiological assessment) is the measurement of penile erection using a penile transducer (usually a circular strain gauge) and a recording instrument. For a detailed description of plethysmography and its use in cognitive/behavioral interventions see chapter 5.

disclosure of additional paraphilias.[5] A nonconfrontive, matter-of-fact approach is usually most effective in lessening denial.

- *The plethysmograph measures behavioral change over time.* The assessment validates the effectiveness of specific behavioral interventions and allows interventions to be "fine tuned" to the resident's needs.

- *Plethysmography allows clients to validate their own progress on accessible charts, fostering a sense of hope and accomplishment.*

Intellectually disabled sex offenders discriminate age, sex, and force among stimuli (primarily slides and audiotapes) used in plethysmography just as well as nondisabled offenders (Steinhauser, 1989). In addition, SSP clients have a higher rate of responsivity to such stimuli, which may be due, in part, to the program's treatment milieu where plethysmograph assessments are considered milestones in treatment. Residents do not consider these assessments aversive but actively seek involvement and show pride in their progress.

Interventions with Limited Application

Individual counseling is used with SSP residents in only limited cases for two reasons: first, the unit milieu, not the individual therapist, is the key change agent for the client; and second, clients with certain character disorders often distort individual counseling by manipulating the session therapist, by misunderstanding the intent of the counseling, or by using the relationship as a power base for impressing other clients.[6] But if a client has treatment needs that cannot be met by the modified therapeutic community or group therapy, he may receive individual counseling with special goals for specific types of disorders.

When individual counseling is prescribed, it is both time-limited and has very specific goals. During the Inhouse phase of treatment, counseling may be prescribed and assigned by the Treatment Team if the client needs more clarification of the group process; needs help fitting into the group milieu (desensitization); or is regressing or grieving. On a case-by-case basis,

---

[5] *Paraphilias* are "recurrent intense sexual urges and sexually arousing fantasies generally involving either (1) nonhuman objects, (2) the suffering or humiliation of oneself or one's partner (not merely simulated), or (3) children or other nonconsenting persons" that are acted upon or obsessively thought about (*DSM III-R*, p. 279). Paraphilias include, among others: pedophilia, exhibitionism, fetishism, frotteurism (the clothed rubbing of the genitals against a nonconsenting partner, usually in a public place), voyeurism, necrophilia (attraction to corpses), zoophilia (animals), coprophilia (feces), klismaphilia (enemas), urophilia (urine), and telephone scatalogia (obscene telephone calls) (p. 290).

[6] Michael Comte of Gig Harbour, WA, who works with intellectually disabled clients, has found it useful to tape the session and have the client listen to the tape between counseling sessions. This reduces distortion and reinforces the content discussed during the session.

clients dealing with their own past as victims of sexual abuse are also referred to the staff psychologist for individual treatment.

Medical interventions are selectively used, subject to the doctor's, Treatment Team's, and client's approval, when other methods do not correct sexual obsessiveness. Low dosages of Mellaril[7] and Depo-Provera[8] are the two medical interventions the SSP uses to control hypersexual behavior; neither has proven to be a magical solution, though low dosages of Mellaril appear more effective than Depo-Provera injections.

Even when medical interventions have been successful, some clients deliberately sabotaged their gains by sexually acting out. These clients stated that when faced with giving up part of their sexuality (becoming impotent and reducing their sexual appetites) they tried to regain it however they could.

The lack of expected success with these medical interventions may be due in part to the SSP's philosophy. Because medical intervention is the most intrusive method of treatment and control, it is the last resort in the SSP; therefore, clients using medical interventions tend to be the most compulsive and least motivated to change.

Card sorts[9] have been useful only as a tool to measure denial; they have not correlated to known histories of offense or measured arousal patterns of SSP clients. Therefore, they are of limited value and are used primarily as references; clients are not confronted on the basis of discrepancies.

Ineffective Interventions

Masturbation satiation[10] has not proven effective with SSP residents because the intervention requires complicated fantasy switching which is

---

[7] *Mellaril* is a phenothiazine antipsychotic drug that decreases aggression and causes secondary impotence as a side effect; it is usually used to control thought disorders and affective disturbances (Barnard, Fuller, Robbins, & Shaw, 1989, p. 80).

[8] *Depo-Provera*, a form of medroxyprogesterone, appears to decrease the frequency and intensity of sexual thoughts/erections/ejaculations and general aggression by lowering the testosterone in the bloodstream to pre-pubertal levels (Barnard, Fuller, Robbins, & Shaw, 1989, pp. 73-74). This intervention is used so rarely that the SSP has not needed to create a consent form; it borrows a protocol and consent form from the CTP Sex Offender Program with staff explanation (for a copy of the protocol and request form, see Knopp, 1984, pp. 303-4).

[9] *Card sorts* provide a "self-report profile of sexual interest" (Knopp, 1984, p. 35). Clients are asked to sort cards describing deviant and nondeviant sexual activities or situations into seven categories ranging from highly arousing to highly repulsive. When combined with plethysmography, card sorts establish an offender's level of denial by contrasting an objective measurement of his sexual arousal with a "self-report [which] often encompasses what [the offender] would like to be true" (Salter, 1988, p. 200).

[10] *Masturbation satiation* "attempts to reduce [deviant] arousal by boring the patient with his own deviant sexual fantasies" (Barnard, Fuller, Robbins, & Shaw, 1989, p. 89). In this technique, the offender first

difficult for the therapist to monitor accurately. Further, there is a growing suspicion among SSP staff that offenders with organic syndromes do not reach sexual satiation easily.

Fantasy and urge logs are generally not helpful to intellectually disabled offenders in monitoring their deviant thinking. Not only are their logs inaccurate, but clients' obsessiveness and urges may increase during periods of intense tracking. In a few cases, tracking fantasies and urges has proven useful when, with staff help, clients catalog deviant fantasies using tally cards rather than rewriting their fantasies as they occur.

For several reasons, the SSP has reduced its emphasis on *empathy training*. Traditionally, programs teach empathy training by showing videotapes of former victims describing the abuse-related difficulties they experienced as children and adults. However, many SSP clients became aroused to such tapes. It appears that intellectually disabled offenders who did not learn empathy skills during their developmental stages may not be able to learn them as adults. Since disabled offenders seem more responsive to the real and possible consequences to themselves than to their victims' difficulties, the SSP teaches offenders to predict what others may be thinking or feeling in a given situation, but does not expect it to have an emotional impact on them.

* * *

While differences in treating disabled and nondisabled sex offenders exist, treatment adaptations for the disabled offender can be made to work successfully. Proven treatment modalities can be creatively and sensitively tailored to take into account the limited reasoning abilities of this population. Intellectually disabled offenders respond to teaching that is concrete, repetitive, and respects their humanity. Many such clients, written off as hopeless by the general public, are able to change their lives and control their offending behaviors as a result of their training in the SSP's comprehensive program.

---

masturbates to a nondeviant fantasy, then switches to a lengthy period of masturbating without ejaculating to a single element of his deviant fantasy, all the while verbalizing his fantasy into a tape recorder. The purpose is for the offender to associate masturbation with the unpleasant sensations of boredom and frustration without enjoying the pleasure of ejaculating.

PART II

TREATMENT COMPONENTS

CASE STUDY

Kevin's Background and Orientation

OFFENSE HISTORY

Presenting Offense

On November 10, 1986, Kevin was arrested and charged with Rape I and Sodomy I[1] of the 12-year-old retarded daughter of his ex-womanfriend. The presentence investigation report stated that Kevin had kissed her on the breasts, had her masturbate him, digitally penetrated and had sexual intercourse with her. The victim was unable to verbalize the events; information came from the victim's 8-year-old brother who had witnessed the assault and from Kevin's confession.

While Kevin originally said he molested the victim in anger to get even with her mother for a specific event, he later admitted that he had abused the girl six times.

Prior Offense

In 1983 Kevin was charged with Rape I, Sodomy I, and Sexual Abuse I with a three-year-old female in a babysitting situation; the charges were later dismissed when the accusers did not appear in court. Kevin denies that any sexual touching took place.

BACKGROUND

Kevin is a 33-year-old white, single male, born in a small town in Oregon. His family is from a lower socioeconomic level. Kevin is the fourth of eight children. There were no apparent medical complications during gestation or birth. He is diagnosed

---

[1] In Oregon statutes, the charge of sodomy does not necessarily indicate anal intercourse; it is used to cover sexual penetration of any kind.

as "mildly retarded." According to Kevin, he was raised in a close-knit family that went to church together every Sunday. While he recalls his childhood as being totally blissful and harmonious, his recollection conflicts with information gathered from other family members and from institutional records.

The family moved often, sending the children to live with relatives or to be wards of the state when times were tough. Kevin's father was reported as often physically abusive toward the children, although Kevin says, "We only got spanked when we deserved it."

Kevin attended special education classes when he went to school. He was explosive, lied to teachers, and stole from peers. He learned only a few math and no reading skills.

At age 14, he and his younger brother were committed to a training center for the developmentally disabled. The two boys had much earlier set fire to a neighbor's house. Kevin claims the fire was accidental; he never realized that the fire was why they were institutionalized. He remained at the training center for four years.

At the training center Kevin continued to be emotionally explosive and to lie. On one occasion he and some "buddies" sneaked into a utility tunnel and destroyed the institution's electrical fire alarm system causing several thousand dollars in damage. As a consequence he was confined in a maximum security cottage.

While at the center he became sexually active with a number of female residents in clandestine liaisons of short duration. According to Kevin, part of the thrill of sex was in getting away with it. Although Kevin adamantly denied having sexual experiences with male peers and often expressed his hatred of homosexuals while in SSP groups, he befriended an openly homosexual resident and demonstrated high sexual arousal to men during an arousal assessment.

At age 18 Kevin was discharged from the training center and entered a group home where he lived for one year. He was discharged for assaulting his roommate (who Kevin says had stolen from him) with a padlock tied to the end of a rope. He successfully completed the two years of probation stemming from this incident and has not reoffended in this manner.

He lived with his parents for a year before he was placed in another group home where he was given Prolixin for hyperactivity. He experienced strong side effects, including visual disturbances and difficulty in walking.

While at the group home he met a retarded woman who lived in her own apartment in the community. He moved in with her and referred to her as his wife. They had a son who was born with abnormalities, including a cleft palate. They brought him home, but the Oregon Children's Services Division removed the child after receiving complaints from Kevin's "in-laws." His wife was placed in a group home and Kevin was not allowed further contact. The relationship had lasted approximately three years. He bitterly blames the woman's parents for the loss of his child and his wife. Kevin says, "This is the hardest thing that has happened in my life."

Work History

For about three years Kevin worked in several sheltered employment jobs. He was considered a hard worker, though extremely task-oriented. He had difficulty working cooperatively with others and did jobs incorrectly rather than admit that he did not understand or could not read simple directions.

He quit work to move home and help care for his mother when she was seriously ill. After three months at his mother's home he began receiving SSI benefits. He moved in with his victim's mother about six months prior to his arrest.

He developed a friendship with a convenience store owner in the neighborhood and worked as a volunteer for him for 20 to 30 hours per week. The store owner reported that Kevin was an extremely dependable worker but was limited in the work he could do because of his poor reading ability.

ENTRY INTO THE SSP

Kevin participated in the SSP for 26 months of Orientation, Inhouse, and Transition treatment and one year of Aftercare.

Orientation

When he was admitted to the SSP, Kevin chose to focus only on developing vocational skills. He was cautious and explosive. He often isolated himself and rarely interacted with peers. A staff treatment goal for Kevin was to get him to view treatment as both safe and possible. To reduce his anxiety and neutralize his fears, a CTT and a peer coach were assigned immediately.

Staff identified no *urgent* treatment concerns (i.e., escape risk, suicide ideation, or assault potential). The Treatment Team approved a standardized Orientation treatment plan (that would later be modified to address his individual treatment needs) and reviewed it with Kevin within 72 hours of his arrival. Within the first month, Kevin began undergoing a series of assessments and evaluations, including psychological and psychiatric/medical evaluations, an educational assessment, a leisure interests and abilities assessment, and a psychosocial history.

Clinical Assessment

Kevin does not appear to be a fixated pedophile with the accompanying obsessive fantasy and masturbation cycle, nor does he exhibit an entrenched justification system to rationalize his actions. His reluctance to discuss events probably is due to shame and may be an indication of an ego-dystonic reaction. Drug or alcohol abuse did not appear to be a factor in the offense.

Five factors contribute to Kevin's sexually deviant behaviors: congenital brain defects, interruptions in his bonding development, blurring in the development of sexual boundaries, a survival mentality, and low self-esteem.

• *Congenital brain defects.* A number of factors indicate that Kevin's brain defect is congenital, including minor physical abnormalities commonly associated with damage of the developing brain, lability of moods, reading and math disabilities, poor muscular coordination, difficulty with spatial perception, grandiosity, and chronic feelings of isolation.

Secondary evidence pointing to genetic brain defect includes a more severely retarded brother who is institutionalized and Kevin's having fathered a son with congenital abnormalities.

Kevin has difficulty in tracking interactions in groups and is easily frustrated and often explosive. He is also rigid, resists changes or new situations, and often initially refuses to cooperate with new expectations. There is no reported incident of head injury which could account for these problems.

- *Disruption of bonding process.* Kevin was born into a large socio-economically deprived family and as a child lived with various relatives due to his acting out at home. His placement at a training center left Kevin quite vulnerable and emotionally needy. He has often become attached to staff, visitors, or peers in an unrealistic way. He has become despondent when these relationships have ended or did not pan out the way that he would like. He is particularly sensitive to perceived rejection and is easily manipulated by those whom he likes.

- *Blurring of sexual boundaries.* At the training center Kevin was exposed to a variety of sexual partners and practices which were premature to his emotional development, resulting in poorly defined sexual interests. During a psychophysiological assessment, he demonstrated significant arousal response to all presented themes, including female and male adults and children, in both consenting and nonconsenting scenarios.

- *Survival mentality.* Kevin developed "street smarts" which allowed him to survive in the community despite his limited intellectual resources. He ingratiated himself to authority figures such as landladies and small business owners in the neighborhood, collected recyclables, and told "white lies" to avoid conflicts. His manipulations and lies have been apparent on the SSP unit from time to time, as well as in the commission of his crime. He does not, however, appear to be criminally sociopathic beyond his personal survival needs.

• *Low self-esteem.* Kevin views himself as "ugly" and "unlovable," causing him to over-react negatively to constructive feedback, in turn preventing him from learning from his mistakes. He sometimes tries to compensate for his low self-esteem by exaggerating his accomplishments to others, a tactic often viewed as obnoxious and grandiose, further impeding his ability to establish relationships with others.

Buying into Treatment

Kevin's CTT carried out a series of interviews with him designed to make Kevin feel that program staff were interested in him and understood his problems. His peer coach explained the rules, introduced him to other residents and staff, and helped him follow the unit schedule for the next six weeks. At the end of that time, the peer coach presented Kevin to the accountability group as a person who was ready to act independently and to assume full resident status and responsibilities.

Soon after arriving, Kevin was assigned to the Phoenix family group and to the Orientation group where living skills necessary for self-care on the unit, the SSP's terminology, and treatment principles are taught. The Orientation instructor was especially chosen for her nonthreatening approach to classes and her ability to engage residents in treatment. She reported that Kevin was very quiet in her groups, rarely participating; was slow to process feedback; and had trouble listening. When he shared his colored pencils with another resident and worked at the same table on a separate project, the instructor saw it as a breakthrough.

[This case study continues with A Review of Kevin's Inhouse Treatment preceding chapter 5.]

4

ORIENTATION

Orientation represents a critical beginning in helping the SSP client feel safe and supported in his new environment.[1] Following a one- to two-week pre-Orientation adjustment period on the unit, the client begins formal Orientation during which his treatment needs are assessed and his treatment-focus areas are identified.[2] Throughout this period staff encourage the client to take ownership of his treatment process, emphasize that he can make responsible choices, treat the client with respect, and act as a reliable sounding board for his concerns. Gradually the client gains a sense of security as he moves from the prison milieu to treatment. He builds self-confidence and begins to feel better about himself as a result of large doses of positive attention. He is encouraged rather than ordered; projects are designed for his particular learning style; and staff model honesty and openness.

During Orientation clients are expected to meet four specific goals: (1) understanding unit rules, routines, and expectations of the program; (2) meeting and becoming familiar with all members of the treatment community; (3) developing a sense of attachment, comfort, and investment in the program; and (4) demonstrating competencies in basic living skills.

Once a week residents meet in an Orientation support group composed of new residents from the two SSP treatment "families" (Cross-Roads and Phoenix). The group is facilitated by a staff member chosen for warmth, sensitivity, and the ability to engage the participants in treatment. New clients may express their feelings about their treatment experience or outside concerns. To build trust with each other, group members make a commitment to keep what is said in the group confidential, and clients are invited to share who they are. The group's main purpose is to strengthen interpersonal relationships and to teach "support for change." After a client "graduates" from Orientation, he is always welcome to come back to this group.

---

[1] See Appendices C & D for graphic representations of the timing and interaction of treatment components.

[2] Treatment-focus areas consolidate clients' treatment issues into five identifiable categories: social skills competencies, medical/psychiatric, alcohol/drug abuse, personality disorder, and sexual deviancy (see chapter 5).

Assessment

The client undergoes a comprehensive assessment and evaluation process, including psychosocial and detailed sexual histories; psychological tests; alcohol/drug, academic, leisure, psychiatric, nursing care, and social skills competency assessments;[3] and documented behavioral observation. Those with positive neuropsychiatric findings are referred to the CTP psychologist for more indepth testing using the Halstead-Reitan battery.[4]

At the end of the Orientation stage, assessment data are tabulated and presented to the Treatment Team to develop individualized treatment strategies in each of the resident's identified treatment-focus areas. All residents are reviewed by the Treatment Team within 10 days of admission, at 30 and 60 days after admission, and then at 60-day intervals for the first year. After that time, Treatment Team reviews are conducted at least once every 90 days until the resident is discharged from parole in the community.

Family Groups

When the SSP accepts the client, he is assigned to a 12- to 15-member *"family" group* (either *CrossRoads* or *Phoenix*)[5] to which he will belong throughout the Orientation and Inhouse phases of treatment. CrossRoads usually includes sexual and other types of offenders; all Phoenix family members are sex offenders. To reinforce the treatment taking place within the SSP, members of the families attend five groups, each meeting for a maximum of 90 minutes. Group names are different for each of the two families in order to promote separate group identities, but clinically they cover identical issues while allowing the flexibility to respond to new issues brought up by different clients.

CrossRoads Family Groups

The five CrossRoads Family groups include Moral Inventory, Solve My Own Problem, Group Issues, Self-disclosure, and Business and Progress.

---

[3] The battery of tests includes Minnesota Multiphasic Personality Inventory (MMPI), Millon Clinical Multiaxial Inventory (MCMI), and Rorschach, if indicated; WAIS-R, Woodcock Reading Mastery Test, Key Math Diagnostic Arithmetic Test, informal interview/self-assessment of learning skills, and Draw-a-Person (DAP). See Resources.

[4] A battery of tests to evaluate brain-behavior functioning. See Resources.

[5] New clients are assigned to family groups as openings occur. Each family group is guided by a Therapy Supervisor who is clinically responsible for the residents' treatment. The Therapy Supervisors have Masters degrees and use consultants as needed. Under the clinical supervision of the Therapy Supervisor are four Correctional Treatment Therapists (CTTs), each of whom has a maximum case load of four residents. One CTT works exclusively with newly admitted residents (supervised by the Aftercare Therapy Supervisor) and may be involved in individual counseling, facilitating groups, designing and conducting

• *Moral Inventory Group.* Facilitated by a Therapy Supervisor, this group holds family members accountable for their behaviors during the prior week in six basic areas: assaults, threats, drug talk, sex/crass talk (sexual joking or swearing), escape talk, and unearned privileges taken. "Other things I have done that I need consequences for" encourages the client to explore with the group personal issues that he may otherwise dismiss. Weekly checks are taken to see whether or not he has been disrespectful when confronted for aberrant behaviors on the unit.

The Moral Inventory Group breaks into smaller groups of five, each led by a member of the leadership group.[6] The Therapy Supervisor moves from group to group assisting in the discussion as members go over their worksheets and give their own evaluations of their progress; the group gives feedback about members' actions. Discussion follows as to "consequences" members must perform, such as writing an essay about their aberrant behaviors, offering apologies, working on the ward, or making collages.[7] Carefully chosen to address each resident's clinical issues, consequences are given for threats, power struggles between clients, noncompliance with rules, or work assignments not completed. Consequences help maintain the group culture and establish behavioral limits. If clients are involved in assaults or sexual acting out, they are returned to prison.

• *Solve My Own Problem (SMOP) Group.* This group is peer-led with staff support. Group work is based on a three-step worksheet completed by the client prior to the meeting: *the problem—how I see it; the solutions—ways I can solve it;* and *the commitment—what I will do.* Several client worksheets are presented and discussed at each group meeting. The CTT evaluates each client's worksheet and gives him written feedback.

• *Group Issues Group.* Group issues are defined as any situation, problem, or concern involving three or more members of the group. Client leaders and co-facilitators construct an agenda for discussion from items of current interest collected during the week. No new items may be added once the group begins. The meeting is peer-led, using an open discussion format.

---

workshops, supervising recreational activities, writing psycho-social histories, conducting alcohol/drug assessments, developing and monitoring treatment plans, and using the penile plethysmograph.

[6] The CTT and the Therapy Supervisor discuss the composition of the leadership group. Then, with group feedback, the Therapy Supervisor makes the final choice based on the clinical needs of the residents (e.g., anti-social or power-oriented residents are not placed in leadership positions). The names of those chosen for leadership are presented to the group for a vote of confidence.

[7] Since self-disclosure is generally difficult for these clients, the act of making a collage, especially one related to a specific behavior, is both a challenge and an activity reinforcing openness and awareness of choices.

• *Self-disclosure Group.* Based on the premise that self-examination is critical to the change process, this group is designed to provide a safe forum for the client to reveal who he really is. Its evolving format allows the group to determine areas to be covered during thorough self-disclosure.

With staff facilitating, residents keep track of who participates. Residents who have successfully completed their own self-disclosure support those who are currently disclosing. To promote group members' ownership of the feedback process and to formally affirm the completion of a "healthy," distortion-free disclosure, group members vote on its quality. Clients may use the following outline as a presentation guide:

— childhood events and your reaction to them;

— your complete criminal history—not only of known disclosures but also of actions you have not yet disclosed;

— criminal thinking before, during, and after your crimes;

— your set-up for victims, how you convinced victims not to tell, or how you bullied victims;

— your reasons for coming to the SSP;

— how you are changing;

— how you are accepting responsibility for your crimes;

— what you are learning about victim empathy.

• *Business and Progress Group.* This peer-directed group handles daily operational problems and procedures, and evaluates clients' treatment plans and job assignment progress. The meeting is divided into two parts: the business group and the progress group. The business segment monitors specific unit procedures and helps the client learn structured ways to deal with day-to-day decisions like borrowing clothes or choosing TV programs. During the second half of the meeting, the progress group alternates weekly evaluations of each client's treatment plan progress and his job assignment performance.

Phoenix Family Groups

Phoenix Family members also attend five groups: Accountability, Sexual Deviancy, Treatment Plan Review, Problem-solving, and Business and Homework.

• *Accountability Group.* Led by the Therapy Supervisor, this primary group maintains the culture of the Phoenix Family using the same issues addressed in the CrossRoads Family's Moral Inventory group, but differs in its approach to consequences. To counter client fears of favoritism and to introduce an element of chance, the Therapy Supervisor assigns consequences using a "drawing card" system to allocate ward work. For example, when the client is to perform so many hours of ward work, he draws a card designating a specific job, e.g., "clean the bathroom tiles." He may draw a "double" card, doubling his ward work. He may draw a card that says "work by yourself," meaning his "buddies"[8] cannot help him; or he may get a "free choice" allowing him to work in any ward work area. Close culture is maintained by allowing buddies to help each other complete the ward work; however, until the work is completed, all buddies' privileges are suspended, encouraging cooperation.

To keep the group functioning smoothly, each week the accountability group also evaluates culture-maintaining jobs such as roll call, wake up, ward-work monitor, confrontation monitor, and activities monitor. In addition, the group monitors the "privilege board"[9] to check any developing patterns of misconduct.

The privilege board system is designed to build cooperation and teach family members "If my buddy loses, I lose." The system's goal is to foster compliance with basic expectations; without such compliance, treatment cannot take place. Every client is responsible for meeting five basic expectations:

- attendance at groups, workshops, activities, therapy sessions, other meetings, meals, taking medications, etc.;
- wake up/room check, i.e., wake up at 6:00 a.m. on weekdays, and clean personal living area for daily inspection;
- a daily one-page journal entry;
- hygiene, i.e., shower, shave, shampoo, and brush teeth before 10:30 a.m.;
- one negative and two positive confrontations with other clients every day.[10]

---

[8] To give each other support and assistance, family members are grouped into "buddy" systems of three or four members according to the bedroom areas they occupy on the unit.

[9] A privilege board system is used in both families with slight variations. For example, in the Phoenix family the privilege board is a chalkboard with a permanent line for each of the 15 family members.

[10] Each resident's list of treatment issues—identified in group by consensus and confirmed by each resident's CTT—is posted in his group room. Negative confrontations relate to treatment issues: when a resident "shuts down" in response to feedback about keeping his living area clean, for example, another client may confront him for that response. Volunteering to help a peer with homework is an example of a positive confrontation.

A "No" is given when the client fails to meet one of these expectations. If one member of the buddy system gets a "No," the others in the buddy system also get a "No."

If a buddy system gets no "No's" for a day, its members earn certain privileges for the next day: listening to their radio, using the telephone, lying on their bed during free time without sleeping, watching TV in the evening. If a buddy system has gone the entire week without any "No's" in a specially selected area (e.g., "room check") then the buddies get late night privileges, including popcorn and late night TV on the weekend.

Clients can earn between four and eight hours of vacation time for the month by meeting all expectations. A client can use his vacation time by requesting time off from the treatment activities for up to one day a month. However, if he gets a "No" the day before his vacation, he can miss the treatment activities but has no other privileges.

• *Sexual Deviancy Group.* This peer-led group provides an open and candid forum for the clients to discuss their sexual deviancy patterns. In a nonconfrontive atmosphere the client learns to evaluate and modify his deviant behaviors, emotions, and thinking.

Because sex offenders give feedback to each other more effectively than a staff facilitator, staff remain outside the group's circle to intervene and give process observations. The group format follows four steps: (1) What did they say you did? (2) How did you get your victim to go along with it? (3) What did you tell yourself to convince yourself that it was OK to do it? (4) How did you get your victim to keep it a secret?[11]

Clients make covert and minimal arousal conditioning tapes (see chapter 5), share their behavioral assessments, and eventually write "clarification letters" to their victims (in which the offenders take full responsibility for their offenses).

• *Treatment Plan Review Group.* At least once a month each client reviews his treatment goals in three main areas: personality disorder, alcohol/drugs, and sexual deviancy. In this peer-led group (with staff help), the client presents his treatment goals, reports how he perceives his progress, and receives feedback from the other group members.

• *Problem-solving Group.* Issues of interpersonal relationships or maintenance that arise during the week come to the attention of this group.

---

[11] Question (1) is asked in this form to circumvent the client's denial. The other questions get the client to begin admitting his deviant behavior and identifying his deviant pattern.

Led by an assigned group leader and using a predetermined agenda and a four-step format, clients thoroughly discuss problems and suggest solutions. The group leader summarizes the situation; group members vote on whether or not to agree with the summary. The next week they have a follow-up discussion to see if the problem is lessening. While not actually solving the clients' problems, the group process allows members to experience working it through. Staff support the group leaders and occasionally point out ways to facilitate the process; they do not offer solutions to problems.

• *Business and Homework Group.* Similar in format to the Cross-Roads Family Business Group, this group provides time during the week to work together on class, group, or workshop assignments. Clients either assist each other or ask for staff assistance.

Workshops

During Orientation the resident attends three workshops which introduce him to this model for learning and form the basis for future learning in the treatment stage: Criminal Self-talk, Personal Basics, and Self-care.

Criminal Self-talk. Offered either in group settings or individual instruction, this workshop uses role playing, collages, art, and videotaping to help residents develop a working familiarity with the SSP's eight different criminal self-talk statements (see Appendix E).[12] Using illustrated worksheets (see Appendix F) as a guide, participants go over these errors one by one. The four basic goals of this workshop are understanding that thoughts precede actions; understanding what self-talk is; learning the eight criminal thinking errors; and identifying and "owning" at least one of them.[13]

When teaching the self-talk concept, the instructor models a basic task (such as drawing on paper) and asks the residents to repeat out loud the instructions used to complete the task: "Pick up the pencil; move your arm to the paper; lean your hand on the edge; press down on the pencil point; move your arm in a curve; lift the pencil from the paper." The task is then repeated. This time the instructor tells the residents not to say the instructions aloud, but "inside their heads." Residents repeat this technique until they realize that self-talk is what they tell themselves about all the things that

---

[12] Adapted from Yochelson & Samenow (1976-77).

[13] While programs for sex offenders of average intelligence use many thinking errors, the SSP focuses on a single primary thinking error for each offender because of its clients' limited reasoning ability and difficulty with memory.

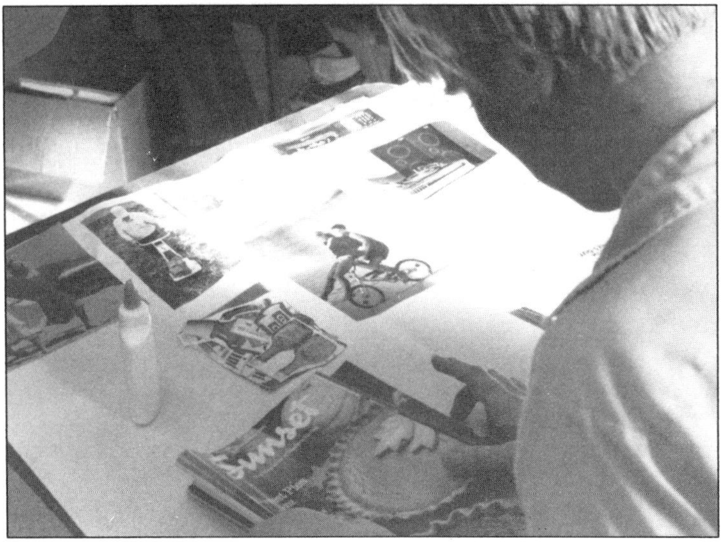
A resident works on his self-talk collage.

happen around them each day; that their self-talk starts upon waking up and does not stop until they go to sleep; that self-talk is what they tell themselves about people, places, or things; and that self-talk can even be about themselves.

Clients often use personally damaging self-talk. In the process of working on his self-concept, one client was able to articulate the way he talked about himself in a rather lengthy self-talk statement: "I am ugly, no woman would ever want to be married to me, I will always be unloved." He discovered that he repeated this statement or its shortened form—"I am ugly"—at least 10 times a day.

One example of criminal self-talk is "Me First," defined as: "I am the best; no matter what I do, I deserve the best, and everyone else is garbage." "Me First," one of the most common patterns of thinking among offenders in the program, is approached in several ways:

• It is identified as a problem. Clients know they can sometimes hide their behaviors from the staff, but other residents cannot be fooled. Therefore, both the client and his peers are part of the identification process.

• The client discusses in a group how he displays "Me First" behaviors.

• He completes projects such as a collage illustrating his typical behaviors.

• In a treatment group the client may "self-focus" on his "Me First" behaviors.

After learning what criminal self-talk is and identifying their primary criminal self-talk statements, residents are prepared for the *Smart Self-talk Workshop* offered in the Inhouse treatment stage, where they learn to re-work their criminal self-talk statement and replace it with a smart self-talk statement. The client mentioned above, for example, reassessed the accuracy of his "I am ugly" negative self-talk and replaced it with his new self-talk statement: "Even though I am ugly, I can still have a girlfriend and be loved." He has lived in the community for seven years and has been married for five years.

Another client countered his incessant talking with the Stop statement, "Shut up, Edgar!"

As these examples illustrate, residents' smart self-talk statements may seem crude and self-deprecatory. But this method succeeds by allowing the resident to develop his statement in his own language. Residents' self-esteem increases as they use their statements to improve social interactions with peers and staff.

Personal Basics. This workshop is considered an activities therapy class, and meets for 12 sessions during the morning activity period. Clients

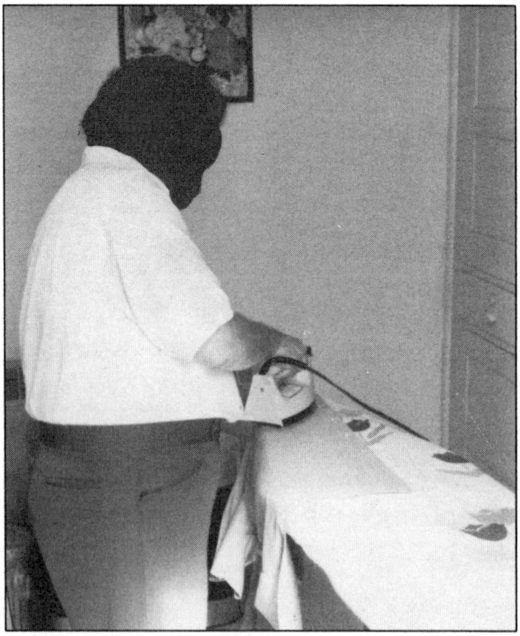

Learning personal basics—ironing

learn how to make simple clothing repairs; use a sewing machine; iron clothes; keep their bedrooms clean; use the telephone; and plan a meal, determining calories, fat, and cholesterol content.

Self-care (hygiene). This final Orientation workshop helps the client develop self-care skills, including how to prevent sexually transmitted diseases. Using a worksheet (see Appendix G), the facilitator assesses the level of instruction each client needs and designs classes accordingly.

Because the Orientation phase is crucial to the client's successful completion of the treatment program, staff use only limited confrontation with the client during this period. Peers and staff determine the feedback approach depending on how much pressure the client can handle. If he has a great deal of anxiety when he first comes to the unit, any confrontive feedback is given only by staff and the client's buddy. Unless the new resident develops an attachment to the program at this stage, he will not be able to withstand the more intrusive approaches necessary to the initial stages of treatment. Efforts to fragment his old established habits and patterns will not be effective, and he might easily give up and return to prison.

CASE STUDY

A Review of Kevin's Inhouse Treatment[1]

Containment of Negative Behaviors

When Kevin felt criticized he often yelled threats at staff and residents, then stomped off. Once he ripped up his journal, saying, "I don't want to do it. I'll just have to burn this place. I have my ways." In another incident he yelled, "Just give me an M-80 and I'll blow this fucking place up! Don't anyone push me or I'll crush heads. So back off and leave me alone!" He could not accept feedback, and his behavior so intimidated other residents, they did not feel safe speaking to him in group.

Kevin's anger problem had to be addressed immediately. Kevin was assigned to assist his CTT in developing a behavior contract that would reward him for responsible behaviors and give negative consequences for threats. The contract specified, for example, that when Kevin became angry, he would excuse himself and go talk to his buddy, or he would take a 10-minute relaxation break. A negative consequence was doing ward work in the hallway with his buddy where everyone could see him. Threatening episodes gradually decreased from three to four daily to two to three per month.

---

[1] This account of Kevin's treatment logically follows a sequential order which could fit nicely into a number of theoretical models, but it would be unrealistic to represent the SSP's treatment program as being this neat and tidy. Although the problems and interventions presented here are accurate, the sequence of interventions is only generally accurate. The uniqueness and inconsistencies of each client require flexible treatment; some interventions had to be repeated as Kevin experienced new situations and stresses.

COMPREHENSIVE TREATMENT PLAN

Personality Disorder Section

Goals:	Date Achievement Expected	Date Resolved
(Problem: Kevin is unable to accept criticism from peers as demonstrated by his yelling and threatening of others.) Increase frequency of listening to feedback without yelling or making threats.		

Methods:

1. CTT will review with Kevin the number of threatening behaviors as reported in the resident daily confrontation log during the previous two weeks.
2. Kevin will begin to self-chart threatening behaviors and making slash marks on his calendar for each incident on a daily basis.
3. Kevin will role-play with a buddy on how to listen to criticism without threatening responses three times per week.
4. One time per month Kevin will make a videotape of three different incidents, demonstrating "old me" (threatening, yelling) behaviors and "new me" (accepting criticism calmly) behaviors. He will show the videos to the group.
5. Journal focus: Kevin is to write about one situation each day when he used his Stop and Go statements to prevent himself from yelling and making threats.
6. Kevin will work with the Recreational Therapist to develop a relaxation technique he can use in stressful situations.
7. At the end of each day, one of Kevin's buddies will debrief him on his successful handling of situations when he was criticized.
8. CTT will instruct Kevin to walk away from situations when he feels he is losing control. He will return within two hours to resolve the conflict.

Treatment Team Leader or Physician ____________________ Date Resident ____________________ Date	Resident Name, OSH #, Unit

Education

After Kevin became relatively stable on the unit, he began a series of experiential workshops on anger management, self-talk, relapse prevention, sex education, and leisure skills, among others.

Kevin struggled in group situations because he had difficulty tracking what was going on in the group and because he was afraid of "looking dumb" in new situations.

He was particularly sensitive about his poor coordination. He often sat away from the group and refused to participate in activities requiring physical coordination. When the Recreational Therapist tried to teach him bowling, Kevin declared, "I have my own unique way of doing things. I will never change it." The Treatment Team decided Kevin should be involved in *noncompetitive* activities and would be held accountable for participating in them. In addition, workshop leaders would encourage him to respond to situations that he could understand where he would not be at risk of "looking bad." He gradually resisted less and became somewhat more open to taking risks.

Participating in academic classes in the SSP's school was a big step for Kevin; upon admission he had adamantly refused to be involved in scholastic activities. He was attracted by having access to the SSP's computer. In school he worked on changing money, telling time, math, and reading skills. Kevin was friendly and cooperative except when frustrated, when he would say, "I don't usually do this" or "I never did this like this in the past" and shut down. On these occasions, the Educational Specialist confronted him for arguing and physically turned her back on him to work with another student. Within minutes Kevin typically apologized and began to ask questions in order to complete the assignment.

Self-knowledge

The next phase of treatment for Kevin involved encouraging his self-disclosure and teaching him self-evaluation. Treatment activities included completing a psychosexual history, participating in a sexual arousal assessment, completing a series of graduated self-focus steps about his deviant behaviors in group, and completing an alcohol/drug assessment with staff assistance and support.

Because Kevin needed to feel that staff acknowledged the physical and sexual victimization in his institutional past, he began individual counseling to explore how his thinking about his victimization had affected his life.

Kevin also participated in group art therapy sessions for 16 weeks. Initially, his artwork reflected his level of comfort at interacting with peers, the group, and the unit. Kevin's first few projects were incredibly closed and constricted, e.g., while working with clay, he built a heavily walled fort. As he progressed in various self-disclosure activities, his work became more colorful and open.

Therapeutic Alliance

Kevin began to develop an attachment and genuine trust in his CTT. When he fell in love with another resident's wife, he tearfully confessed it to his CTT and asked for her advice. While previously he had steadfastly maintained that he was going to live in the woods as a hermit after treatment, he began expressing a stronger commitment to change and began talking about his plans for Aftercare. The Treatment Team formalized his decision by having him, his CTT, and the Director sign a contractual agreement specifying such aims as, "I am going to continue not being around children; when things get tough, I will ask for help; and even though I feel scared, I will share what's going on with me with others." This "fostered dependence" was viewed as healthy; his willingness to ask for help increased Kevin's chances of making a successful transition into the community.

Self-help

Treatment began to focus on building competency. Treatment plans called for Kevin to demonstrate such skills as risk taking, making assertive requests rather than aggressive ultimatums, progressive relaxation, using *Stop* and *Go* smart self-talk statements, and sexual arousal control.

Kevin's *Stop* statement in this focus area was, "Look at yourself." His *Go* statement was, "They have the right to do it their way." While observers might regard these statements as irrelevant to his treatment issues, SSP staff experience shows that the *content* of the statements is less important than their symbolic meaning as labels in the self-confronting ritual.

Kevin was trained in covert sensitization as a way to control his deviant sexual arousal. His participation followed his usual pattern: initially he was extremely resistant, but as he developed comfort and skill he became adept and committed to the process, eventually helping to train other residents.

Kevin's Monday Schedule

6:30	*Wake up* and take care of personal basics
7:15	*Breakfast*
8:00	*Housekeeping, wardwork* (the ward is cleaned by residents). Room checks for cleanliness are made by resident monitors.
9:00	*ATs.* Activity Therapy led by the Recreational Therapist. Leisure and recreation activities are taught; today, Kevin—along with his buddy and seven other residents—attends a circuit fitness class where he'll work out on a rowing machine and a stationary bike, lift weights, and do exercises to increase his flexibility.
10:00	*Group.* Today is Accountability Group, addressing disruptive behaviors on the unit. It is often a highly stressful meeting for Kevin, because he is repeatedly confronted for threatening people.
12:00	*Lunch*
1:15-2:30	*School.* Kevin is working on math skills. He has trouble working with a peer tutor so works with the Educational Specialist. He really enjoys working on the computer.
3:00-4:30	*Workshop.* Alcohol/Drug Workshop, "Family Ties." Staff teach basic concepts using experiential activities and help residents apply the information to their own lives. Kevin's project is to produce a collage of the roles of his family members and his role in relationship to them.
5:00	*Dinner*
6:00-6:30	*Canteen.* The unit canteen is open twice a week for the residents to buy snacks, cigarettes, etc.

(continued)

7:30-8:30	*ATs*. Passive card and board games. Kevin likes to play "Sorry" and Dominoes with one or two other residents.
8:30-9:00	*Journal*. Kevin writes of his day, treatment issues, etc. He is assigned a "journal focus" of "Two times I got angry today and how I handled it responsibly." Due to Kevin's poor writing skills, a buddy helps him write it and then Kevin copies it over.
9:00-9:30	*TV*
9:30	*Lights out*

Kevin's Tuesday Schedule

6:30	*Wake up* and take care of personal basics.
7:15	*Breakfast*
8:00	*Housekeeping, wardwork.*
9:00	*ATs.* Kevin again goes to his circuit fitness class with other residents.
10:00	*ATs.* Gardening class. Kevin particularly enjoys gardening because he likes the physical nature of the work and because he can work alone.
11:00	*Free Time.* Kevin often uses his free time to do wardwork or help others do theirs. He likes sweeping, mopping, and waxing floors.
12:00	*Lunch*
1:00-2:30	*Anger Management Workshop.* Kevin works on his Stop statement ("Relax") and his Go statement ("Try"). Kevin's individualized assignment is to self-chart his anger outbursts.
3:00-4:30	*Workshop.* Alcohol/Drug Workshop, "Family Ties."
5:00	*Dinner*
6:00-7:30	*Group.* Sexual Deviancy Group. Kevin is working on making a full statement of what he did. He's having a very hard time talking about it and sometimes walks out. Later on, making covert sensitization tapes helps him with his disclosure.
7:30-8:30	*SA.* Sexaholics Anonymous meets on the unit at this time. Kevin has not yet been approved to participate in this outside group, so he uses the time to do his self-charting for Anger Management class.
8:30-9:00	*Journal*
9:00-12:00	*TV.* Because Kevin and his roommates met all expectations on Monday, they have earned "privileges" to stay up later than the usual 9:30 lights out.
12:00	*Lights out*

[This case study concludes with Kevin's Transition Treatment preceding chapter 6.]

5

INHOUSE TREATMENT

During the Inhouse treatment stage the entire treatment community focuses on issues wherever and whenever they develop; thus, treatment in the SSP is a 24-hour process. Because of the self-defeating behaviors of most of its clients, treatment is goal-oriented and individualized. Clients learn to label their thoughts and behaviors as "old me" and "new me," and to internalize these new self-perceptions as they work in any of five treatment-focus areas identified during Orientation. Change comes about with the help of the modified therapeutic community in conjunction with group and activity therapy and the selective use of individual counseling. Psychoeducational classes stress anger management and cognitive restructuring.

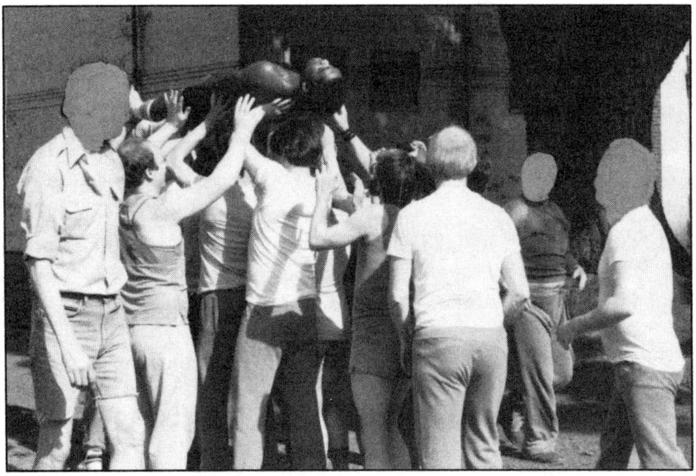

Learning trust, working together in activity therapy

Treatment Techniques

Treatment techniques include *behavior contracting, daily journal writing*, and *self-charting* by residents.

Behavior Contracting

In *behavior contracting*, the resident and his CTT write an agreement incorporating into his treatment plan clear and detailed behavior expectations and goals related to his specific treatment issues. Making the resident a primary participant in development of the contract reinforces his internal locus of control[1] and permits him to take ownership of his change process. The contract ritualizes the concept of commitment, saying to the resident, "No more excuses. You have outlined your own choices. Now it is your choice to live up to them." He has the opportunity to show whether he has the character and will to stand up to his word, to achieve goals, to be a success.

Residents often write goals that are unrealistic. Character-disordered offenders have grandiose expectations of themselves or set unrealistic goals because they feel that is what the therapist wants. Working on the behavior contract in group as well as in individual counseling and requiring the Treatment Team's approval help the resident set realistic contract goals so the resident can accomplish *something*, no matter how small. Residents first write a goal for the next 10 days; then 30 days; finally 90 days, unless intermediate goals are more appropriate and achievable. After approval, the contract is posted in the unit for all residents to see. Residents demonstrate that they have achieved their goals through projects, speeches, videos, collages, and so forth.

For example, John, who is working on alcohol and drug abuse issues, wrote, "I'll never take another drink," as his first goal. With group and staff help, John broke that goal down into the intermediate goals he needed to accomplish, e.g., "I will find out how alcohol affected my father," a goal that was less threatening to him and increased his awareness. A few of John's other intermediate goals included discovering what stood in the way of his being sober; learning how he could have fun if he did not drink; and figuring out how to handle other people making fun of him for not drinking.

Daily Journal Writing

The *daily journal*, used by all residents during all phases of treatment, is a daily written log of self-talk and/or behavior. As in behavior contracting, the resident and the CTT define the journal focus for a particular treatment plan. A resident's journal focus might be to identify three conflict situations during the day and to outline how he resolved them. For a more basic journal focus the resident might write down three things he accomplishes each day or three conflicts he is able to walk away from

[1] Traditionally, a *nonoffender* intellectually disabled population receives frequent overt reinforcement, e.g., "You're doing a good job." The SSP uses less overt reinforcement, e.g., staff ask a client, "How do *you* think you're doing?" Staff then evaluate the client's self-evaluation. If he says he thinks he's doing well, staff ask, "How does it feel to *you* to do something well?", rather than saying, "Yes, we think so too."

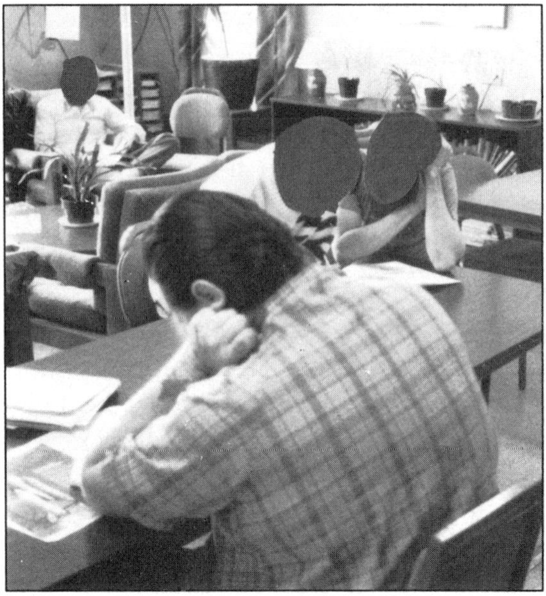

A resident who can't read or write gets help from a buddy in daily journal writing.

without verbally exploding. A resident's journal focus might also be what he is thinking at a specific time during the day, for example, at noon in the dining room while eating. He reviews what he wrote, identifying his criminal self-talk statements by their labels. The journal focus is approved by the Treatment Team and must be clear, concise, and within the academic abilities of the resident.

All residents write in their journals at specific times each day and turn them in at the end of the day for the CTTs to review and comment on their content and focus (not their writing or spelling). If the resident is not abie to read or write, he dictates his daily journal to a buddy. After the buddy writes it down on a separate piece of paper, the resident copies it into his own journal. This transcribing process enhances the clients' reading and writing skills without formal academic instruction, strengthens the buddy system, and increases their sharing about their behaviors and thoughts.

Self-charting

In *self-charting* the resident targets a particular behavior for change, monitors his own behavior, and graphs his progress on a unit-posted chart. This self-control cognitive strategy increases the resident's awareness and his monitoring skills. His improved self-awareness and ownership of the task promote responsibility, increase his independence, and develop his internal locus of control. The resident's prior training in targeting behaviors and the staff's initial reinforcement for his accurate self-evaluation are important.

The more proficient the resident becomes at identifying and charting his treatment progress, the more effective the strategy is in involving him in his own treatment.

"A New Me"

The resident is encouraged to work in all of the treatment-focus areas identified at the completion of his orientation stage so that he can become a totally new person, acquire a new identity, become a "new me."

Ted's and Martin's examples below illustrate the concept of developing a "new me" identity as an integral part of personality and behavioral change:

> Ted is a sadistic rapist with a long institutional history and third-grade reading and math skills. He was physically abused as a child by his stepfather and carries a lot of rage which comes out in vindictive behaviors towards other residents. Because of the abuse and his institutional experience, he is fearful and suspicious.
>
> Ted was given a number of projects to help him deal with his old vindictive self. They seemed to have little impact, but Ted did not give up. When an art therapy intern worked with him, Ted began to express his emotions in art, a less verbal approach that slowly broke down his resistance. Through various media, Ted was able to express some of his rage, making his "old me's" vindictiveness visual. He began to accept the part rage played in his deviant pattern.
>
> In journal entries and collages, Ted focused on his "pay back" behaviors ("old me"). For one project, Ted wrote and illustrated how he tried to hurt others. His journal focus, which became the center of his counseling with his CTT, was outlined as follows:
>
> (a) Who I thought about hurting today.
>
> (b) How I was going to hurt them.
>
> (c) How I stopped myself from hurting them.
>
> On Sundays Ted will read back over his week of journal entries and draw/paint the feelings that he had the past six days.
>
> * * *
>
> Martin, a pedophile, was assigned to interview 10 residents and staff over a 90-day period on how a well mannered person acts. After each interview

he was to write an essay about what he had learned from the experience. He reviewed these essays with his CTT for further feedback. During the same 90-day period, Martin was to read a simple book about "friendships," which also became part of his discussions with his CTT.

For a separate project, Martin presented a series of collages depicting his feelings of superiority ("old me") to his treatment group once a month for four months. Martin explained his "old me" in which he thought of himself as better than everyone else, and presented his "new me" in which he accepts his weaknesses and those of others. The group gave Martin feedback about how his presentation came across and about ways he had shown his "old me" and "new me" in the past few weeks.

TREATMENT-FOCUS AREAS

Significant change in the resident's behavior is only possible through a holistic treatment approach to his dysfunctions. Key to this approach is the SSP's multidisciplinary Treatment Team. Its task is to integrate the client's work in any or all of five treatment-focus areas: social skills competencies, medical/psychiatric, alcohol/drug abuse, personality disorder, and sexual deviancy. The Treatment Team and the resident develop specific goals in each of these areas.[2]

Treatment-focus planning concentrates the team's attention on the client's problem areas. The individualized treatment plan allows the resident to develop his "new me" within the treatment-focus areas of his choice, even when he chooses to work only in one or two focus areas rather than in all the areas in which he may need treatment. There is almost always at least one element of each treatment-focus area that the client does not resist working on, giving the SSP a "foot in the door" to changing his thinking and behavior.

If and when he completes the treatment goals in his chosen areas, the resident can then choose to work in other treatment-focus areas; if he declines further treatment, he is returned to his parent institution as having successfully completed treatment in the areas he was willing to address.

---

[2] For an example of a treatment plan in one treatment-focus area, see A Review of Kevin's Inhouse Treatment preceding this chapter.

Treatment charts, similar to medical records in psychiatric programs, are kept in the staff office for staff use only. These charts are divided into five sections, one for each treatment-focus area. The treatment goal is the same in all five focus areas: to identify and discard the "old me," and to develop new thinking and behaviors—the "new me."

The explanation of treatment-focus areas that follows makes it appear a more compartmentalized, orderly process than the reality of its application. In practice, all clients get some treatment in all treatment-focus areas (regardless of which areas they initially choose to work on) because of the unit's total involvement in workshops and projects and the constant feedback from buddies and group members. The spill-over treatment effect from client to client is built into the system by design.

Social Skills Competencies Treatment-focus Area

Social skills competencies work is integrated into all other treatment-focus areas; work on survival skills begins in Orientation with personal hygiene, using the telephone, and developing leisure skills, and continues through Aftercare with classes in cooking, using community resources, and individual training in apartment living. It includes all programming, from anger management and problem solving to disputing thinking errors, alcohol/drug treatment, and relapse prevention.

An important part of social skills training is preparation for getting and keeping a job. Wardwork and on-grounds work (see chapter 6) train clients in work responsibilities, job evaluations, and dealing with authority figures.

The goals of the social skills treatment-focus area are to remediate the basic living-skill deficits of the "old me" and to develop competencies for the "new me." As in other treatment-focus areas, six primary elements are used to teach these skills: the modified therapeutic community, "family" treatment groups, individual counseling, leisure classes, academic classes, and workshops.

The Modified Therapeutic Community

The entire treatment unit is transformed into a 24-hour-a-day instructional laboratory. The facility is organized and decorated with workshop-generated material (e.g., a "Push Your Own Buttons" banner from the Anger Management Workshop) to focus on a specific theme, reinforcing the main points being taught through all elements of the environment.

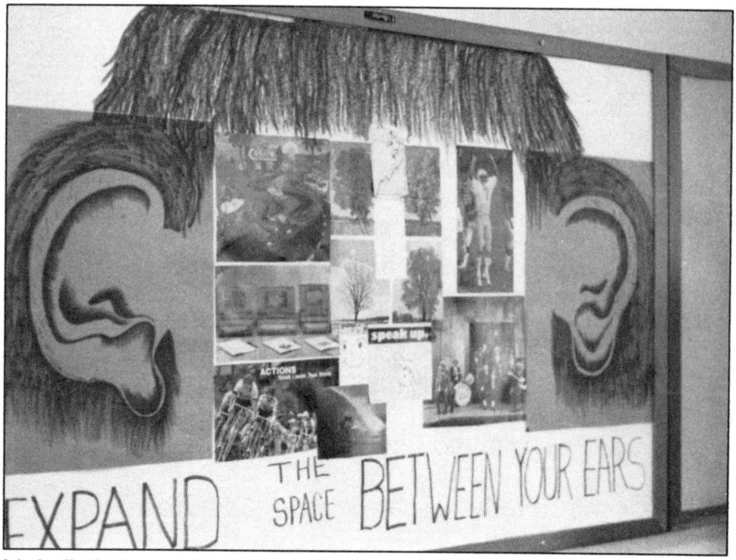

This bulletin board shows how the whole unit is used to illustrate a theme.

"Family" Treatment Groups

The five "family" treatment groups each resident attends use experiential approaches in developing social and interpersonal skills, assertiveness, and problem solving.

Individual Counseling

Individual counseling focuses on specific treatment problem areas which are particularly uncomfortable for a resident to deal with in group settings. Using an experiential approach whenever possible, counseling typically focuses on sexual identity confusion, unresolved feelings towards parents, grief counseling, and alleviation of chronic abandonment depression.

Leisure Classes

Leisure classes are an important element in the SSP's therapeutic recreation program (see Appendix H for a description of the recreational activities delivery system), and are central to the treatment delivery system. The impact of prescriptive activity therapy cannot be over-emphasized. Interventions are immediate and powerful. During activities it is difficult for residents to mask their pathologies. Therefore, activity classes are often one of the most effective forums for spontaneous intervention and demonstration of change.

The SSP dedicates 15 hours a week to structured activity therapy classes under the direction of the Certified Therapeutic Recreational Specialist. All treatment staff, not just the Recreational Specialist, conduct

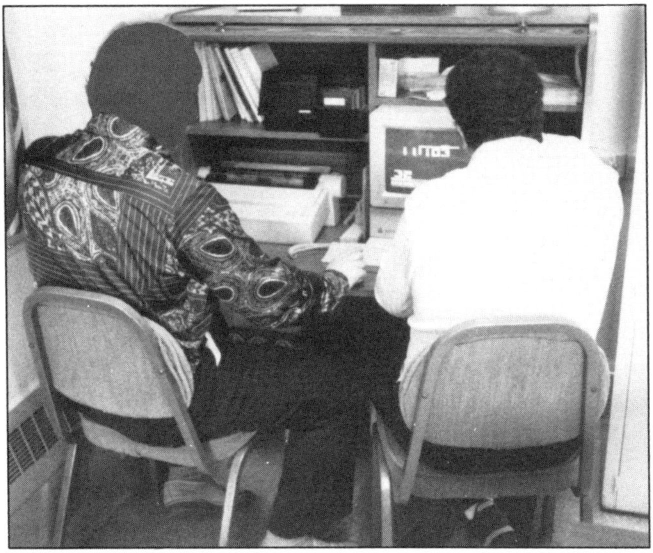

Residents can learn on the computer in academic classes.

leisure skill classes, an expansion of traditional therapy boundaries that provides a more holistic view of the residents and enhances the continuity of their treatment. Classes are prescriptively designed to help the residents develop and maintain social support systems and improve skills which they can later use in their transition to the community.

Academic Classes

Academic classes in basic skills that can be applied to daily living (reading, math, spelling, etc.) are limited to six voluntary participants, and are taught by the Educational Specialist in three 90-minute sessions per week. Students work individually in topic areas of their choice. They can receive help with their work from the teacher, peer tutors,[3] and volunteer student-intern tutors. Modes of instruction include workbooks, flashcards, games, and a computer. The atmosphere of the classroom is relaxed, supportive, and noncompetitive.

Other basic application skills, such as telling time and changing money, are taught to small groups in a workshop format. A variety of nontraditional materials and approaches, including designing bulletin boards, playing games, and computer work, are used to teach these skills.

---

[3] Peer tutors are chosen by the Treatment Team with the recommendation of the Educational Specialist based on diagnosis: a resident diagnosed with Avoidance Personality Disorder, for example, may be assigned to tutor reading. Thus, tutoring becomes a valuable interpersonal learning experience for the tutor as well as an academic growth experience for the student. In some cases, a resident with poor basic academic skills is intentionally assigned to tutor another resident. Working together, both learn at a faster rate.

Workshops[4]

Workshops are the core of the information delivery system and are divided into three categories. Initially, the SSP overextended itself by attempting to develop workshops to meet *all* the needs of the residents. Experience showed that certain key concepts needed to be emphasized and repeated; these became the *standardized* workshops. *Nonstandardized* and *transitional* workshops were developed to meet the evolving needs and interests of the residents.

Standardized workshop topics include *Smart Self-talk* (cognitive restructuring), *Anger Management, Sex Education*, and *Sexual Myths*. These workshops provide a foundation of values and skills necessary for change to occur. All residents participate in the classes which meet in 90-minute sessions twice a week for eight weeks. Each topic is repeated every six months so a resident may be involved in the same workshop several times during his treatment period.

Smart Self-talk. This core workshop begins with a review of the eight basic criminal self-talk statements learned by the resident during Orientation. He identifies which of the eight statements his criminal self-talk is based on. A *Stop* statement is then developed to be used as an intervention mechanism in stressful or dangerous situations. The *Stop* statement is balanced with a replacement *Go* statement. For the resident the *Go* statement acts as an escape from a conflict or high-risk situation. For example, when others are pushing him in order to get ahead in line, one resident uses the *Go* statement, "It is okay to let others be first." This client practices this self-talk by letting others go before him three times every day, waiting to be last to get his medications. In this way he is reminded at least three times every day to practice his smart self-talk.

Below are some examples of *Stop* and *Go* statements designed and practiced during the workshop. While these statements may seem irrelevant to the treatment issues of the client involved, SSP experience indicates that the content of the statements is less important than their symbolic meaning as labels. Clients use these phrases ritually to interrupt their own negative behaviors and thoughts (like using a mnemonic device). The fact that the statements are in their own words is equally important. Statements are revised as clients continue in treatment.

---

[4] All workshops are based on cognitive restructuring approaches, modifying techniques outlined by Donald Meichenbaum (1977).

Stop: Do I hear the jail door starting to slam shut?

Go: They have a right to do it their way.

These statements were developed by a sex offender who is very afraid of jail and has a hard time viewing a situation another way. His *Go* statement constantly reminds him that others' points of view may be valid.

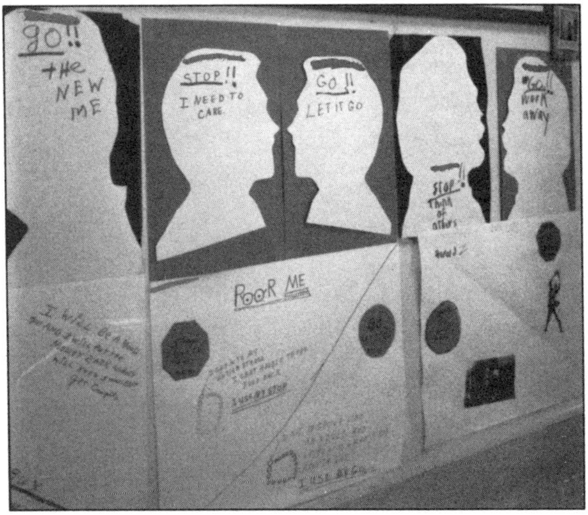

"Stop" and "go" bulletin board

Stop: Your thinking is stupid.

Go: Be responsible.

These two statements are from an antisocial sex offender. His *Stop* statement means that even his best thinking has gotten him in trouble, resulting in his being in prison. His *Go* statement is a shorthand reminder that irresponsibility has marked his past.

Stop: I need to care.

Go: Let it go.

This example is from an alcoholic, mentally ill pedophile who cared for no one but himself. When he wants to take advantage of others, he first uses his *Stop* statement as a reminder of his "new me." He then uses his *Go* statement to let go of the grudges he uses to justify hurting others.

To retain the residents' attention for 90 minutes the workshop periods are divided into four basic parts: warm up, object lesson, and individual and group activities. Following is an example from one of the first

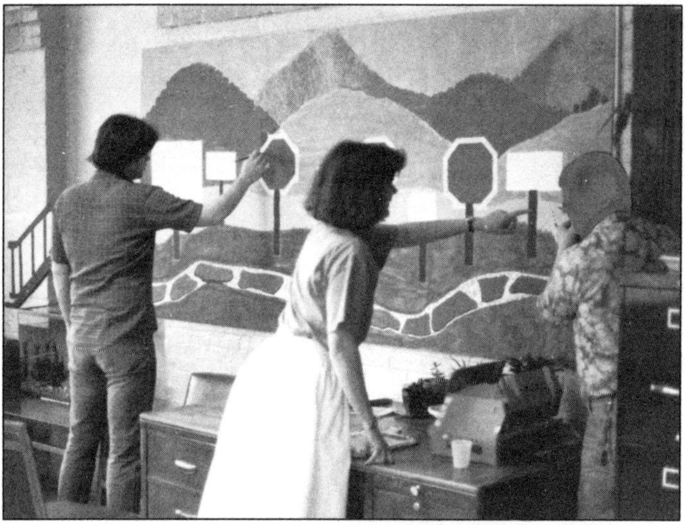

An art therapy intern helps residents with their "Stop" mural.

lessons used in the workshop. Suggested plans are accumulated and filed for future use by the next team of workshop leaders.

> ***Warm up:*** In the previous lesson the residents each had the chance to identify with a number of cartoons representing the eight thinking errors used in the SSP (see Appendix F). In this session each resident acts out the character he identifies with from the previous lesson. The other residents guess what his criminal self-talk is.
>
> ***Object lesson:*** One of the facilitators shows the group a half-full glass of water and asks them if they think the glass is half full or half empty. The facilitator explains how their positive or negative thinking about the glass of water affects their behavior.

The major time in the 90-minute workshop is given to "fun, interesting, or bizarre" individual and group activities.

> ***Individual activity:*** Each resident is given a picture of a half-full glass of water and asked for a positive statement and a negative statement about the glass.
>
> ***Group activity:*** The residents pair off. Each resident does a large drawing of his criminal self-talk. He discusses with the other person what he is thinking when he uses this criminal self-talk. Drawings can be presented to the larger group if time permits.

Below are other ideas that have been used to emphasize the principles of the Smart Self-talk Workshop.

• An Oregon Highway Department *stop sign* was given to the SSP. Each client traces around it on stiff paper and prints his *Stop* statement inside the outline. The sign is placed on the ceiling above his bed so that the last thing he sees at night and the first thing he sees in the morning is his *Stop* statement.

• *Stop* and *Go* statements are printed on *campaign-type buttons*. Each client wears his button wherever he goes during the entire workshop.

• The Oregon Highway Department built a full-sized, timer-operated, working *traffic light* for the unit. Whenever the red light appears clients go to the nearest person and recite their *Stop* statements. When the green light appears they share their *Go* statements.

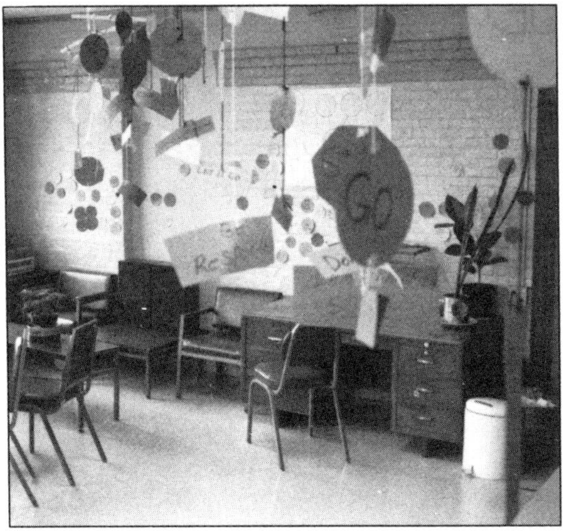

"Stop" and "Go" mobiles hang in rooms and hallways.

• *Mobiles* hung in the group room, the hallway, and in the bedrooms spell out the *Stop* and *Go* statements.

• *T-shirts* illustrating the *Stop* and *Go* statements are worn on workshop days and other times as desired.

• In a mock *judge-and-jury trial*, including prosecuting and defending "attorneys," each client is tried by his peers on how well he uses his smart self-talk. To emphasize the importance of practicing and using smart self-talk, "convicted" defendants face such sentences as: "Before and after each group meeting you must say your *Stop* and *Go* statements;" "You must wear your *Stop* and *Go* shirt for seven days in a row and the shirt must be clean at all times;" "You must interview 10 people about the value of using your *Stop* and *Go* statements." This activity is a powerful reminder that if clients do not use their smart self-talk they will end up in court again.

• Each client develops a *laminated card* the size of a credit card, placing his *Stop* statement on one side and his *Go* statement on the other.

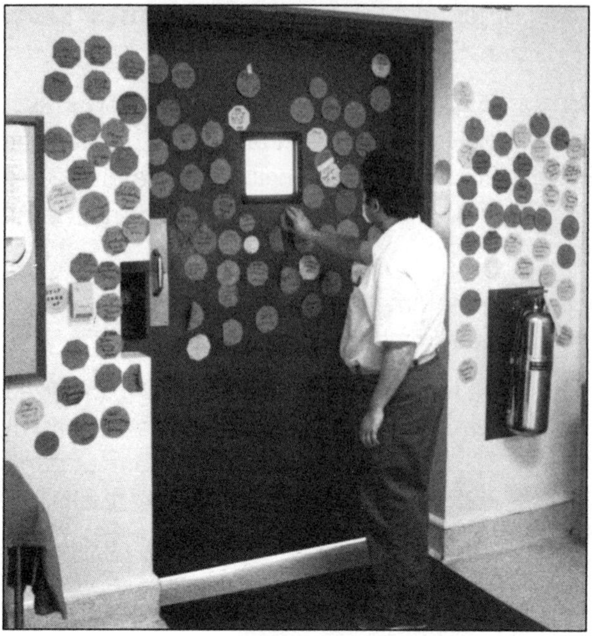

A hot spot for using "Stop" and "Go" statements

The unit's telephone number is also on the card so the client can call for support from outside the unit when he is released on parole.

- A *room tour* is used as a warm-up exercise during the workshop. The entire workshop visits each member's room to see how he displays his *Stop* and *Go* statements. The clients explain what their statements mean.

- Each client makes *"wall buttons,"* a stack of small colored paper *Stop* signs and *Go* lights bearing his statements. When the client successfully uses one of his statements, he tapes his button on the wall or door nearest the location of his success. Clients and staff can easily see the areas of frequent conflict.

Instead of rewarding residents with methods based on an external locus of control (as in token economy systems), the Smart Self-talk Workshop emphasizes the value the resident receives from controlling his behaviors.

The workshop group may develop a "wrap-up" game, skit, or song to demonstrate what they have learned. Skits and role plays are videotaped for future reference. When they complete the workshop, the residents receive certificates of recognition. At the closing ceremony, the group shares refreshments they have made.

The constantly evolving Smart Self-talk Workshop is repeated twice a year to give residents extra exposure to these important concepts.

Anger Management. The Anger Management Workshop is similar in basic format to the Smart Self-talk Workshop and is as important in the overall treatment program model. Its two primary goals are for the resident to become familiar with six anger management skills, and to be able to identify and develop a competency in one of them: (1) disputing (cognitive restructuring); (2) acceptance (learning about his handicap and having a more realistic expectation of himself and his abilities); (3) listening; (4) assertiveness; (5) stress management (relaxation skills); and (6) escape/avoidance (learning how, when, where to remove himself from anger situations).

The Anger Management Workshop is conducted for eight weeks, with two 90-minute sessions per week. Each session is divided into two parts: the first half of the workshop consists of staff and small-group demonstrations and presentations; during the second half, the participants break into smaller groups of clients who are working on the same competency skill. Each small group has a staff facilitator. The small groups plan and carry out presentations demonstrating a skill they have acquired. Because the emotion of anger is complex and has multiple etiologies, and because no single approach is effective with intellectually disabled offenders, a variety of materials and methods is used, including role plays, video productions, games, and demonstrations, among others.

As in other workshops, Anger Management emphasizes the "old me—new me" theme. The first two sessions focus on the "old me": residents keep a daily anger log to identify the key situations that "push their buttons" and allow them to act out. The remaining 14 sessions focus on the "new me": using a wide range of experiential activities, residents learn new anger management skills and develop "new buttons" they can push to keep themselves in control. After completing the workshop, residents present their projects demonstrating competency (new buttons) in dealing with their anger. Examples of some of their creative projects are listed below:

- Small groups decorate a room to bring attention to their assigned competency. After several weeks of work, residents invite staff, peers, and outside guests to tour each room.

- A magnifying glass is used to demonstrate how anger becomes larger when focused on.

• In triads a speaker gives an opinion to a responder; the responder repeats the opinion word for word, summarizes the opinion, and tries to guess the speaker's feelings; the third person rates the accuracy of the responder. The three residents rotate their assignments and repeat the process.

• A resident attaches a balloon to a tire pump and asks the other workshop participants to give examples of old self-talk. With each example air is added to the balloon until it explodes.

• Working on the theme "push your own buttons," each resident identifies "old buttons" and draws them. He identifies a "new button" he can push during anger-provoking situations. Residents wear these buttons and invite staff and peers to ask questions about them.

Sex Education. This workshop focuses on traditional topics for a sex education course: anatomy, birth control, sexually transmitted diseases, intercourse, and homosexuality. Caring and partner responsibility are emphasized in discussion of all topics. Teaching methods are similar to those used in other workshops, and, as always, material is presented in humorous, bizarre, and dramatic ways.[5] Information is presented in the form of a game show modeled after "Wheel of Fortune"; a humorous movie with a serious message, Condom Sense,[6] is shown; and visits by celebrity sex experts "King Condom" and "Dr. Ruth" (as impersonated by staff and residents) enliven the proceedings.

Sexual Myths. This workshop focuses on common misconceptions about sexuality. Based on the book Male Sexuality (Zilbergeld, 1978), the following myths are discussed and disputed:

- Men should not express certain feelings.
- All physical contact must lead to sex.
- Sex equals intercourse.
- A man always wants and is always ready for sex.
- Sex is a performance.
- A man must orchestrate sex.
- Sex requires an erection.

---

[5] For example, to ensure that all clients knew how to use condoms, the unit held condom relay races using ceramic penises residents had made in a crafts class.

[6] See Resources for film availability.

- Good sex is increasing excitement terminated only by an orgasm.
- Sex should be natural and spontaneous.

Again, a wide variety of teaching modalities is used, for example, small group discussions, movies, computer-generated banners, and the creation of the fictitious character "Robo-Stud."

Medical/Psychiatric Treatment-focus Area

If the resident has any medical/physical problems (Axis III, *DSM III-R*) they are identified during Orientation, and goals and methods are outlined for a treatment plan to be monitored by the psychiatric nurse. Similarly, goals and treatment methods for any identified mental/emotional problems (Axis I, *DSM III-R*) are under the direct supervision of the program psychiatrist. Both specialists implement and monitor the comprehensive medical/psychiatric treatment plan.

Counseling and crisis intervention by the psychiatrist, chemotherapy, and educational modules are the three major treatment components in this focus area. The psychiatric nurse conducts educational modules to teach clients the purpose and side effects of their medications and how they can take responsibility for managing their mental illness. Also taught are basic health education, sex education, AIDS prevention, and first-aid skills.

Alcohol/Drugs Treatment-focus Area

The intellectually disabled offender's alcohol and drug abuse is often overlooked or receives minimal attention in traditional treatment programs. All the impulse control techniques the offender can learn are worthless when his judgment is impaired by alcohol or drug use. Therefore, this focus area commands considerable SSP resources and is considered of primary importance to the success of treatment. Goals for this treatment-focus area are for residents to become sober and maintain their sobriety in the community.[7]

To change residents' abuse of alcohol or drugs, the "old me—new me" treatment approach uses three primary elements: psychoeducational workshops, an inhouse AA group, and modeling sobriety in high profile ways.

---

[7] Due to clients' lack of judgment and poor impulse control, *every* SSP resident is encouraged to abstain from alcohol and street drugs regardless of whether he is diagnosed as alcohol- or drug-dependent.

Psychoeducational Workshops

In two 90-minute sessions per week for a period of six weeks per workshop, SSP residents focus on developing a new (sober) identity, new understanding, new culture, new skills, and new self-talk in seven workshops: Responsible Me, What Happened, How It Works, Walls and Doorways, Family Ties, H.A.L.T., and Stinking Thinking.

Responsible Me. This "new identity" workshop explores self-image, how to change from the outside in. Residents investigate all aspects of "fitting in" as sober adults and learn to identify a label that suits them as new, sober, recovering persons.

After two weeks the workshop has a "recovery party" to mark the beginning of the client's "new me" as an abstainer from alcohol and drugs. A film, *Seventeen and Going No Where*,[8] is also presented. Clients make collages picturing what a sober adult looks like, what he wears, the kinds of job choices he makes, the kinds of friends he has, and the types of recreational and leisure activities in which he engages.

What Happened. This "new understanding" workshop teaches clients the effects of various chemicals on the body, emphasizing how alcohol and drugs make their handicaps worse. It introduces the concept of addiction as a disease and educates clients on the effects of drugs and alcohol on motor control and judgment—including the hazards of drunk driving. This cognitive process uses worksheets (see Appendix I), films and videos, demonstrations, and group exercises to inform in a way that is both fun and dramatic.

In one exercise clients make life-sized tracings of their bodies, drawing the internal organs, then discuss and illustrate the effects of alcohol and drugs on the various body parts.

How It Works. This "new culture" workshop, a primary tool in alcohol/drug treatment, consists of ongoing instruction in AA/NA/Al-Anon programs and philosophies. Designed to help the client attend AA meetings in the outside community, it is the introductory meeting for AA. Clients are introduced to AA's 12 Steps and 12 Traditions, and learn how to act in meetings, how to find a sponsor, how to use the telephone to get support between meetings, and how to attend social functions. The unit holds a weekly registered AA meeting for graduates of this workshop.

Walls and Doorways. Residents are helped to establish their "new culture" in this workshop by reviewing the barriers to sobriety they will face

---

[8] See Resources for film availability.

in the outside community. Using a game-show format with a staff member as host, clients are divided into three or four teams. The teams draw from a collection of high-risk situations and prepare role plays about escaping from them. Scoring is based on team effort: the better a team works together in preparing and presenting the role play, the better it scores in the game. The group as a whole then votes on which team did the best job on the role plays. Scores are kept; at the end of the workshop each team is recognized and the winning team receives a grand prize.

Family Ties. In this "new culture" workshop, residents explore roles in the dysfunctional family. They identify their own roles (then and now), and look at some common ACOA (Adult Children of Alcoholics) characteristics. Clients identify the "search for the enabler," common to substance abusers. The roles presented—enabler, dependent, hero, scapegoat, lost child, and mascot—are visualized, videotaped, and presented to the group. The film *Soft Is the Heart of a Child*,[9] is also used.

H.A.L.T. (Hungry, Angry, Lonely, Tired). In this "new skills" workshop (a relapse-prevention module), residents identify key parts of their relapse cycles, especially "set-up" situations and options for dealing with them. Using role plays, clients act out situations they may face in the community, including alternatives to drinking or abusing drugs.

Stinking Thinking. This "new self-talk" workshop pinpoints justifications, excuses, euphoric recall,[10] and denial self-talk, and helps residents identify the types of self-talk that give them the go-ahead to use alcohol/drugs. Fantasy control is also dealt with through thought-stopping and replacement self-talk.

High Profile Sobriety

Another important characteristic of the drug- and alcohol-free "new me" is *high-profile sobriety* reinforced by the entire modified therapeutic community. In addition to workshops and unit AA meetings, staff model their commitment to sobriety by not wearing clothing advertising or promoting alcohol and drug use, by discouraging the telling of alcohol and drug "war stories," and by sharing their own struggles with alcohol and drug use.

---

[9] See Resources for film availability.

[10] Euphoric recall is remembering only the "high" feelings, and not the hangovers, loneliness, expense, humiliation, and other consequences of drinking.

Personality Disorder Treatment-focus Area

Background

The existence and treatment of personality disorders in the population identified as intellectually disabled are often ignored. Intellectually disabled offenders with serious personality disorders must be clearly diagnosed so that specific treatment programming can be designed to address their deviant behaviors. This treatment area focuses on the distorted thinking behind the deviant behavior, a concept advanced by Yochelson and Samenow (1976-77). They suggest that the "criminal" acts irresponsibly because of the way he perceives and experiences the world; he thinks external events make his criminal actions inevitable. Before his behavior will change, the offender's pattern of thinking must change to include taking responsibility for his choices.[11] This is as true for the intellectually disabled offender as it is for the nondisabled offender.

Three of the offender's key thinking processes must change before his behavior changes: power-thrust (see Appendix J), victim stance, and equating "I won't" with "I can't."

Power thrust. Samenow defines *"power thrust"* as a reaction based on a fear of falling into a "zero state," losing the self. The payoff of a power-thrust is excitement and an adrenalin rush from feeling superior. When the offender perceives failure in any behavioral or cognitive endeavor, he feels dumb and embarrassed—powerless, in the "zero state." The staff's treatment role is to help the resident see things in stages, to point out again and again that one learns from one's mistakes.

The same sense of powerlessness occurs when the offender feels he is being criticized, or is afraid even the smallest thing might go wrong. Again, the offender is given feedback that criticism is something from which to learn. Staff ask him to see whether his expectations were in error or unrealistic from the beginning. The common focus is on having the offender become aware of his cognitive distortions as in the following example:

> George had been a group leader for about a year and a half. He was removed from that position by the Treatment Team to take off some of the pressure so he could concentrate on his sexual

---

[11] In addition to the thinking distortions that Yochelson & Samenow outline, Ross, Fabiano, & Earles (1988), suggest that deficits in social intelligence also play a part: "Many offenders have not progressed beyond an egocentric stage of cognition and are unable to understand the behavior, thoughts, and feelings of other people." These offenders therefore have major deficits in interpersonal problem solving. "These deficits are not in general intelligence—in IQ, but deficits in social intelligence—in the ability to understand other people and the ability to deal with interpersonal conflicts and adapt in a pro-social manner" (p. 30).

> deviancy treatment. George experienced the change as a put-down and a loss of power. He became sullen for several days and didn't know what to do. He protested, "I don't care that I am no longer the leader, in fact, I am relieved to get rid of that job." But residents and staff observed his attempts to regain his power base by increased confrontations with other clients, loud arguments with peers, refusing to comply with parts of his new treatment plan, and making long observations in group sessions about how the new group leaders were not doing their jobs well. His power issues were focused on in a treatment group. As he regained some of his lost status, his affect improved.

Victim stance. "Victim stance" is defined as a state in which the offender manages to defend himself and blame society as unfit. SSP staff and residents label this thinking error "Poor Me." When the offender is in a victim stance, the staff accept no excuses, continuing to focus on the offender, his choices, and their consequences, as in Sheldon's case:

> Every morning the residents' rooms are inspected by a peer. To keep the system honest, these inspections are occasionally double-checked by a staff member. One morning Sheldon, who had been passing inspection without a hitch for weeks, was "caught" by the staff inspection. He blamed the staff for his loss of privileges for that day. He saw himself as a victim of the staff member: she was out to get him, he thought. He saw himself as innocent. Staff helped Sheldon process how he distorted this experience. He was asked to examine how he used this kind of thinking to justify his sexual deviancy and other irresponsible acts.

"I won't" equals "I can't." In the third thought process, the offender translates *"I won't"* into *"I can't,"* repeating this error so often that he begins to think and believe "can't" is the truth, the reality. Characteristically, this stance is ingrained in the intellectually disabled offender; because of his many failures he resists taking any perceived risks.

Staff approach this problem also by not accepting any excuses for the resident's not completing his task. Though the intellectually disabled person has real fears because of his past failures, the personality-disordered offender who says he "can't" do something is really making a statement of refusal. One of the common ways that SSP clients use this distortion relates to their voluntary status in the program:

> A client left behind a radio belonging to the program. Several other clients expressed interest in having it in their rooms. Eventually, Sam accused Frank of manipulating the system to get the radio for himself. Frank's feelings were hurt. He reported to staff, "I can't stand the way Sam is always accusing me." After attempts at problem-solving, Frank decided that he would not deal with the problem—it was too much for him. He would rather go back to prison. His "I won't" (deal with this problem) turned into such a strong "I can't" that he gave up his place in the program rather than change it.

Treatment Goals for Personality Disorder

The client initially works on disrupting his distorted thinking, identifying his "old me" by:

— accepting responsibility more often for present and past behaviors when asked by staff and peers;

— identifying behavioral and cognitive characteristics of his "old me";

— identifying the *central characteristic* of his "old me" in interpersonal conflicts;

— increasing his awareness of the consequences of his behavior on others;

— verbalizing choices more often when upset;

— reducing his feelings of fear, anger, or grief from past life events.

During this part of treatment, the resident feels great frustration, since his thinking (and therefore his behavior) becomes ego-dystonic. His old methods of dealing with life issues are no longer functional and do not provide the "high" of feeling all-powerful. His feelings of attachment and dependency on the program conflict with his sense of frustration.

As the resident gets better at identifying the characteristics of his "old me," he is introduced to the process of identifying "new me" characteristics. Treatment emphasizes the sense of empowerment the client will feel by reproducing these new characteristics. All aspects of treatment reinforce these new behaviors and instill a sense of responsible power and control over his own life. Treatment focuses on helping the client develop his "new me" by:

— identifying, developing, and practicing the behavioral/cognitive characteristics of his "new me";

— learning how to bond in interpersonal relationships;

— becoming competent in relapse coping skills;

— generating concrete future plans.

The primary treatment approach presents the offender with realistic situations requiring him to make choices without emotional investment by staff in the outcome. Low-level confrontations by both staff and peers draw attention to what the resident is doing and the choices he is making; the resident looks at his options and their consequences. When confronting the resident, the staff respect and recognize his capacity and right to choose for himself. The approach is adapted to his particular personality disorder: a more confrontive approach with an antisocial personality, a less confrontive one with an avoidant/dependent personality.

The interventions are ongoing within the treatment milieu. The staff use positive reinforcement for prosocial behavior and thinking: honesty, empathy, effort, identifying and making responsible choices, and pointing out "criminal thinking" and behaviors in other residents. Staff use compliments, recognition, and prescriptive socializing with residents[12] as primary reinforcers rather than the usual token economy system which reinforces the external control commonly used with intellectually disabled offenders. Even in behavior contracting, where the focus is more specifically on behavioral change, the reinforcements are camouflaged in order to foster the resident's ownership of his own rewards.

In prison, struggles over the choice of TV programs often result in violence. As a major social outlet for intellectually disabled sex offenders, TV becomes a vehicle for treating clients' distorted thinking. Both the content of the shows and the process of selection provide opportunities to reinforce treatment.

Residents chosen as TV monitors watch their peers' reactions to TV program content. When a resident reacts inappropriately (e.g., cheering at trickery or dishonesty), the monitor intervenes by debriefing the resident at the conclusion of the program. If the resident is not receptive to this

---

[12] At debriefings, staff are alerted to increase social contact with the client. Without using overt reinforcements, they spend time socializing with the client who has demonstrated responsible behavior. Staff validate the client's "new me" behavior by saying, for example, "That must have felt good to you." They reward clients' efforts toward responsible behaviors with higher-profile, self-reinforcing responsibilities.

discussion, the issue is taken up with his treatment group. Staff do not intervene directly, but, when necessary, may coach the resident monitor.

The SSP teaches clients to clarify their values around TV. Clients make judgments about "good and bad" TV programming.[13] "Good" TV reinforces the treatment values of responsible living, caring for others, and other such ideals. "Bad" TV programming contains sexually explicit or aggressive images, glorifies taking advantage of people, or supports criminal behaviors.

Limited TV viewing is used prescriptively; it is considered a privilege, not a right. If a client does not meet basic expectations, he does not get to watch TV. Resident monitors review the scheduled programs. They ensure that only the scheduled shows are viewed, confront inappropriate client behaviors during the program, and change inappropriate to acceptable programming.

Sexual Deviancy Treatment-focus Area

The inpatient phase of the SSP focuses on three primary sexual deviancy areas: *arousal control and cognitive restructuring, appropriate relationship development*, and *maintenance*. Transition treatment (see chapter 6) concentrates on assisting clients to apply these skills and methods for preventing relapse in an open setting.

Arousal Control and Cognitive Restructuring[14]

Arousal control and *cognitive restructuring* are so closely integrated in their application that they are considered together here. Arousal control encompasses both the use of *plethysmography* in the behavioral laboratory and the cognitive restructuring approaches incorporated in various *cognitive/behavioral interventions*. (Programmatic elements discussed elsewhere—e.g., Criminal and Smart Self-talk Workshops and the Relapse Prevention group—also incorporate cognitive restructuring approaches to controlling deviant sexual behaviors.)

Penile Plethysmography. Research literature supports plethysmography as "the most objective, reliable, and valid means for assessing deviant sexual arousal ... [allowing] direct calibration of penile erection" (Stein-

---

[13] The selection of TV programming follows specific guidelines that give treatment value to the process. On Tuesday, the TV monitors meet and schedule TV for the following week. Each group reviews the schedule and may veto any programs that they feel are clearly against the majority's treatment. The TV monitors meet with the group leaders on Friday to re-schedule for vetoed TV shows. If errors are made in the TV listing, the TV monitors, together, may substitute programs with the staff shift leader's final approval. Any TV show may be shown as long as there is treatment group approval.

[14] The techniques described in this section are *adaptations* of standard procedures for a specific population. Their proper use requires specific training and supervision.

hauser, 1989). While there are some limits on the reliability and validity of this assessment technique, no other assessment procedure consistently separates sex offenders from nonsex offenders (Murphy & Barbaree, 1987).

Before being assessed, each resident is fully informed about the procedure and its possible benefits and risks, as well as possible alternatives and their limitations. He understands that his other treatment will continue even if he chooses not to participate in the behavioral therapy laboratory sessions. If he chooses to participate, the resident also understands that if he has any adverse reactions to the various interventions, the SSP will provide corrective treatment. This information is contained in consent forms written at about fourth-grade level (see Appendix K) and is reviewed both verbally and in writing with the client.

Because fear of the technology, feelings of invasion of privacy, and performance anxiety are potential barriers to valid assessment, residents are desensitized to the assessment process: first they become familiar with the behavioral laboratory and equipment; the Behavioral Therapist (BT) and other residents describe the assessment for the resident; and the resident eventually controls the assessment process in trial runs. Sometimes unrelated counseling sessions are held in the lab to ease a client's discomfort with the environment. The actual physiological assessment begins once the Treatment Team considers the resident psychologically prepared. The client's baseline assessment is completed within six months of his admission and compared to his indepth psychosexual history.

During his introductory laboratory assessment session, the client views an explicit sex-education video while wearing the circular strain gauge around his penis. With paradoxical intent, the BT explains that the client is merely getting used to the gauge and that arousal is not expected during this session. Arousal invariably occurs and is reviewed with the resident as evidence that he is competent and ready for assessment even though staff had not expected it. With this process, the client is successful in demonstrating arousal in the laboratory without experiencing the performance anxiety often accompanying initial assessments.

The baseline assessment takes place over three or four days. In sessions lasting about 90 minutes, the client privately places the strain gauge on his penis and observes both deviant and nondeviant stimuli using slides, videotapes, and audiotapes.[15] The offender is asked why he is or is not

---

[15] Slides of deviant sex acts are kept to a minimum. Videotapes depicting deviant sex acts have been eliminated because some clients reported new deviant fantasies afterward. While audiotapes are not as

aroused to the stimuli and to estimate the ages of the subjects and his perceived level of arousal. To give the client as much privacy as possible the BT records all measurements and comments (see Appendix L) in a separate room. Throughout the session, the client is asked about his emotional comfort.

Slides are used in the first session; in the remaining sessions audiotape descriptions of appropriate and deviant sexual themes are presented. At the end of each session, the client is asked to masturbate while still wearing the gauge until he has reached full erection (without ejaculating). For comparative purposes, the highest recording reached is considered to be 100 percent arousal. Over 95 percent of SSP clients demonstrate arousal levels over 20 percent[16] to some presented sexual theme in the laboratory.

After each assessment session the BT asks the client how he feels. When necessary, the BT initiates specific interventions, which may include scheduling additional debriefing sessions with the client, encouraging him to spend time with a buddy experienced in lab techniques and the assessment process, and/or arranging individual counseling for the client with his CTT. If the client reports a compulsion to masturbate with deviant fantasies, he is instructed to masturbate only to appropriate themes.

After all the data and information are recorded (see Appendices M & N), the Treatment Team and the BT develop individualized behavioral treatment strategies for the client. The resident is reassessed periodically and treatment strategies are continued or modified by the Treatment Team. Only a limited number of clients are assessed during any one period, so that any resulting sexual acting out or aggressiveness on the unit can be closely monitored.

Cognitive/Behavioral Interventions. To address clients' sexual deviancy, the SSP uses four primary cognitive/behavioral interventions: *Minimal Arousal Conditioning, Covert Sensitization, Assisted Covert Sensitization*, and *Aversive Behavioral Rehearsal* (see Appendix O for informed consent forms for these techniques). Client goals for these interventions include:

- early recognition of and control over deviant arousal;
- increasing openness and acceptance of his sexual problems;

---

effective in discriminating sexual interests, clients do not report new deviant fantasies associated with their use.

[16] The generally accepted level of validity is 20 percent (Laws & Osbourn, 1983, p. 314)

— awareness of the consequences of any future deviant acts to himself and potential victims;

— generalizing negative consequences to new situations and to new offense set-ups;

— increasing confidence in himself as a responsible citizen skilled in avoiding sexual problems.

Minimal Arousal Conditioning teaches clients early recognition of their sexually deviant arousal and how to intervene effectively in their patterns. While nondisabled offenders write detailed descriptions of various deviant *fantasies*, intellectually disabled offenders describe *actual events* they found sexually exciting. The interviewer takes notes and helps the offender recall details.

Based on the interview, the BT writes a script which the offender reads or recites with the BT into a tape recorder daily. He sniffs ammonia fumes whenever he is aware of arousal and then begins to read the script from the beginning again.[17] Occasionally a client cannot complete the fantasy because he is aroused repeatedly at a certain point in the script, and his arousal is not decreased by sniffing the ammonia fumes. To prevent a build-up of frustration over what he may perceive as his "failure," the client is instructed to continue the story despite his arousal and to continue sniffing ammonia until his arousal decreases.

These 30-minute daily sessions are supplemented in the laboratory once or twice weekly. The client reads or recites the script while being monitored on the penile plethysmograph. The BT instructs the resident to sniff the ammonia whenever he begins to show any arousal. To enhance the client's ownership of his treatment and to maintain the therapeutic alliance between client and therapist, the BT does not administer any aversive agents.

Covert Sensitization teaches clients the consequences to themselves from their sexually deviant acts, helps them recognize set-up situations, and demonstrates how to use avoidance tactics. Clients are taught to make audiotapes containing the following elements:

— a brief description of a situation that led to an offense (due to their difficulties in sequencing and in following a storyline, clients

---

[17] Inhouse clients use small bottles filled with ammonia-drenched cotton. While off-unit, Pre-release/ Aftercare clients carry ammonia capsules for convenience and privacy. Capsules are preferred for house use as well but the cost is prohibitive.

with lower intellectual abilities are instructed to use short descriptions of the set-up scenario);

— the offender shouting "STOP!";

— some categorical disputing statements he has previously learned in the Smart Self-talk Workshop: "Where has this gotten me before?" "I don't need this, look away." "It's not worth it!";

— a list of all of the consequences that happened as a result of past offenses and the possible consequences of a future offense;

— a statement of what he will do to avoid the situation, for example, "I get off the bus at the next corner. I walk to the nearest pay phone and call my sponsor at 555-1765. I explain to him what I am feeling."[18]

These five steps take about five to seven minutes and are repeated for 30 minutes daily using a tape recorder (60-minute tapes—30 minutes per side—make timing simple). To help the BT and the client know how much progress is being made, the offender reports his own fantasy scenarios in weekly laboratory sessions. Intellectually disabled offenders may require more initial training, particularly when they cannot read: they recite after a BT or listen to a tape recording until they can repeat the script entirely from memory. The protocol for using this procedure is the same as for other cognitive/behavioral interventions (see Appendix O).

Assisted Covert Sensitization is a combination of Covert Sensitization and Minimal Arousal Conditioning, with an additional emphasis on appropriate sexual fantasy development. The protocol is the same as for other behavioral/ cognitive interventions (see Appendix O).

The client records treatment tapes privately, and reviews them with his BT. The tapes are similar to those used in Covert Sensitization, with two differences: the client begins the session with a previously learned relaxation exercise; and at the end, he describes an appropriate alternative sexual outlet to use in a fantasy congruent with his "new me." The scenes are three to five minutes long, repeated for at least 15 minutes a day.

Once the client masters the skill of making tapes, he begins twice-weekly laboratory sessions. During the laboratory session he listens to audiotape recordings of deviant fantasy situations similar to his own, sniffing ammonia when he feels any arousal. The BT informs the client if the client

---

[18] This element is reinforced and expanded on in a later Relapse Prevention Workshop.

begins to get aroused and is not aware of it. When not in a treatment session, the client wears a rubber band on his wrist and snaps it when he feels the urge to fantasize deviantly.

Aversive Behavioral Rehearsal can be a powerfully emotional, intrusive intervention and is used by permission of the Treatment Team only when other modalities do not work. As with all cognitive/behavioral interventions, the client gives his thoroughly informed consent (see Appendix O).

Aversive Behavioral Rehearsal cuts through the offender's minimization and reluctance to talk about the details of his offense and paints a clear picture of the amount of force used. The SSP resident acts out an example of his crime with a mannequin (talking about his thoughts and feelings all the while) in a scene that is videotaped and shared with client-selected peers and staff.

Because a powerful negative emotional experience is associated with the sex offense, making the tape and sharing it are aversive in themselves. Staff take a neutral or supportive approach while the tape is being made, since staff confrontation during the process could damage the therapeutic alliance.[19] Staff and peers chosen by the resident view the tape and give him matter-of-fact feedback on their feelings about the offense, followed by counseling.

Appropriate Relationship Development

The lack of sexual interest in mutually consenting adult partners is more often due to social anxiety than to the absence of urges (Schwartz & Masters, 1983). Therefore, lowering the level of social anxiety by desensitizing the SSP resident has proven a more effective treatment approach than *Appropriate Arousal Conditioning*, a method used with nondisabled sex offenders.[20]

Desensitization occurs through social interaction assignments with peers, staff, and student volunteers. Assigning topics that are not related to sexual feelings appears to decrease clients' anxiety during social contacts

---

[19] This approach differs from the usual application of the technique used with nondisabled offenders. Traditionally, Aversive Behavioral Rehearsal is used confrontationally to break down the offender's emotional and cognitive distortions and to focus on their harmful effects.

[20] Traditionally, Appropriate Arousal Conditioning teaches clients to masturbate to appropriate stimuli. But it is questionable whether masturbation to pictures carries over to increased interest in human subjects for intellectually disabled offenders. Further, such training may lead the intellectually disabled offender to frequent pornography outlets in search of sexually explicit photographs after being released into the community, an activity that could quickly lead to reoffense.

with adults and to increase their arousal (as measured in the behavioral therapy lab) to appropriate sexual themes.

SSP staff have observed many clients unable to develop appropriate relationships with adult females prior to treatment, who have sustained such relationships after graduating from the program. Staff have found no other, more convincing explanation to account for the change than the desensitization that takes place on the unit.

Maintenance

After the client has demonstrated the ability to control his deviant arousal through the use of cognitive/behavioral interventions, he enters the maintenance phase. He makes one or two tapes weekly using Minimal Arousal Conditioning, Covert Sensitization, or Assisted Covert Sensitization; his progress is monitored by his BT with new arousal assessments every three to six months. If his ability to control his deviant arousal diminishes significantly, the client repeats whichever treatment mode is most effective for him.

Since SSP residents, like all incarcerated Oregon offenders, have determinate sentences, they are treated for transition into the community at large. Chapter 6 details the ways in which the client maintains work in his treatment-focus areas while shifting some attention to learning and rehearsing specific community-survival skills.

CASE STUDY

Kevin's Transition Treatment

Pre-release

Kevin's self-esteem, based on his identity as a good worker, provided a solid support base for beginning his transition into the community much earlier than most residents—after about a year of Inhouse treatment. Because his therapists felt he would benefit more from a task-oriented work situation than from the groups he had such difficulty understanding, he was allowed to work part-time in the Oregon State Hospital kitchen. He proved to be a very hard worker whose efforts were greatly appreciated by the kitchen staff. A problem developed when some of his co-workers from the Women's Correctional Release Center got him to pass messages to inmates.

As he felt more successful in his kitchen work, he began to discount the importance of other treatment assignments. At one point, his therapists suspended him from the kitchen to help him reorder his priorities.

Transitional residents met weekly to plan outings and activities that would be likely to carry over to their lives in the community. True to his pattern, Kevin initially resisted and declared the outings a colossal waste of time. Again, he became more tolerant of these activities as he became more comfortable with them.

Before entering the Aftercare component of the program, Kevin developed a relapse prevention plan identifying the places, people (e.g., the SSP as "home base" and his Aftercare buddies), and activities (e.g., the YMCA for sport and exercise, an adult hobby club for model car racing or ham radio operators) Kevin needed to communicate with in order to maintain his "new self." He identified thoughts, feelings, and situations he should avoid to prevent relapse. He additionally developed and memorized an intervention plan to use when he found himself in a vulnerable state.

Kevin's Crisis Card

(Front of card)

Problem:	Argues, Threatens, Assaults, Easily led, Sexual deviancy
Set-up Feelings:	Dumb, Abandoned, Strong sexual urges.
Set-up Situations:	Babysitting, Criminal friends, Too much free time, Being friendly with children.
Set-up Thinking:	"Poor me, I need it. They want it."

(Back of card)

Help/Action

1. Stop Statement: "STOP, I don't need deviant sex!"
2. Walk away.
3. Use covert sensitization disputing.
4. Go statement: "I need to talk to someone."
5. Return to the unit.

Emergency Plan:

SSP #: 555-1923 SA Meeting #: 555-6941 Crisis Line #: 555-2060

IF I RE-OFFEND, I WILL TURN MYSELF IN RIGHT AWAY.

Parole Office #: 555-9357

The Treatment Team gave Kevin a temporary leave three months before his parole date in order to allow him to live with another Aftercare client. He continued working at the OSH kitchen and attended evening groups. With this structure, the SSP had the option of pulling Kevin back into Inhouse treatment as needed. Just before his parole release he began working in a sheltered workshop; upon release he again received SSI payments for his living expenses.

Maintaining Responsible Identity in Aftercare

After Kevin began Aftercare he transferred to a food services training program at a sheltered workshop. Within two months he was placed as a part-time baker's assistant in a local grocery store. He worked 20 hours a week and continued to draw SSI benefits. Following an on-the-job training period, he was allowed to bake donuts without supervision. After ruining several batches, he was suspended from work for a day. He then tearfully admitted that he did not know when the oil was ready because he could not read the temperature gauge on the fryer. Marks were then placed on the gauges so he could see the correct temperature.

Kevin developed a relationship with a woman who undermined his relapse prevention plan when it interfered with her needs. She insisted he spend time with her while her children visited on weekends, and Kevin chose to do so. Once she left him to babysit her children, and Kevin chose to stay with them. This situation was eventually considered a violation of Kevin's parole, and he spent a week in the county jail. While he was in jail, his womanfriend developed a relationship with an SSP dropout she had met through Kevin.

When Kevin was released, he was in a state of agitated depression. He asked for help from the SSP and attended daily debriefings on the unit and weekly activity outings. When encouraged to attend support group meetings in the community, he declined because of his continued frustration in trying to understand group dynamics.

Kevin's employers were willing to keep him on because of his good job performance in the past, but they warned him that they would not be so tolerant in the future.

While in Aftercare, Kevin bought a bicycle, found an adult bike club, and began to attend its outings as his primary leisure activity. Because of his poor coordination, lack of physical conditioning, and after several minor accidents, he decided not to join the group. This experience was regarded by staff as a beneficial experiment for Kevin in making choices, a breakthrough in risk-taking.

He began collecting cans for recycling, saving enough money to buy a C.B. radio so he could listen and talk to truck drivers. He made friends at a local truck stop, where he met a mentally ill woman dishwasher with whom he struck up a relationship. She was older than he and had grown children. After three months he moved in with her at a low-income apartment. Her mental illness forced Kevin to extend himself to meet her needs as well as focusing on meeting his own, breaking up his tendency toward self-absorption. Eventually, they married and he began to feel a part of her family. The relationship has been stormy but viable. The couple joined a fundamentalist church and began attending socials and occasional Sunday services.

Aftercare treatment and parole were completed in one year. Kevin continues to visit the SSP from time to time, particularly during times of marital crisis.

Prognosis

If Kevin can maintain his strong community support system and follow his relapse plan, he stands a good chance of not reoffending. Ongoing mental health counseling would enhance his ability to maintain himself responsibly in the community. If his support system should deteriorate, leaving Kevin to his own resources, he is highly likely to get into another inappropriate relationship, a situation that could easily lead to a reoffense. Explosiveness will always be a problem for Kevin. However, with his newly acquired intervention skills, he should be able to keep his problem behaviors from becoming destructive.

6

TRANSITION TREATMENT

Making a successful transition from treatment in the SSP to fully independent community living is the ultimate goal for all residents.

This third and final stage in the SSP treatment process occurs in three phases: (1) an inpatient phase, including applying for admission to the Pre-release/Aftercare program, transition planning, and Pre-release/Aftercare groups; (2) the transition process, including redefining the client's relationship to the unit, parole planning, early discharge, and later post-release; and (3) graduation.

Inpatient Phase

Beginning with Orientation, every treatment plan review aims at the resident's transition into the community at large. Although transition is a crucial part of SSP treatment, that focus can easily be lost in an intensive inpatient milieu. Thus, the Therapy Supervisor, acting as a consultant and program designer, maintains the transition focus throughout all treatment plan reviews by concentrating on improving the resident's basic living skills in self-care, prevocational training, use of leisure,[1] education, and related social areas.

Because their basic living skills are frequently inadequate for fully independent living, the resident's functioning level is matched with the most suitable type of Aftercare living/working situation. The longer clients live in the community with Aftercare support, even when it is a struggle, the more likely they are to develop comfortable social niches and the less likely they are to reoffend, as Richard's example illustrates:

> Richard had been in and out of institutions for a number of years. He viewed institutions as safe providers for his basic needs and would commit nuisance crimes or threaten suicide in order to come to the attention of the authorities. He often became upset when SSP staff would not assume responsibility for keeping his pack of cigarettes,

---

[1] To counter the tendency of intellectually disabled clients to isolate themselves, the SSP requires each client to develop a hobby or other leisure activity skill and to find and join an adult group promoting that hobby or skill: e.g., model car racing club, bicycle club, citizen's band radio operators group, bowling league.

> doing his laundry, and personally inviting him to scheduled activities.
>
> The first time he began Aftercare in the community he was afraid of failing and ran away to another state where he previously had been committed to a state hospital. He was returned to Oregon as a parole violator, and eventually he returned to the SSP. His treatment plan was redesigned to focus solely on his integration into the community. After one year in the community, he continues to adapt to the varying demands of responsible living despite several lapses.

Applying to the Pre-release/Aftercare Program

Nine months prior to release, a resident submits an application to be considered for the Pre-release/Aftercare program (see Appendix P). The Treatment Team conducts a full review of the resident's treatment methods and progress since his admission. Team members evaluate his amenability to Pre-release/Aftercare programming, the amount of time left in his original sentence, his compliance with program rules, and the presence and strength of community support systems in his Aftercare plan.[2] At the end of the review, the Team decides whether or not to accept him into this phase of treatment.

If the resident is not accepted for the SSP's Pre-release/Aftercare program, he has two alternatives: he may be returned to his parent correctional institution and released through its transitional planning unit; or he may be released directly to his home community with SSP assistance. If he is to be released through prison transition, staff help the client develop a release plan which he can implement with the assistance of the correctional release service unit. In cases where the client has an established support system of family and friends or mental health services already in place, he is released directly to his home community. The SSP helps the client to connect with community mental health organizations, to secure housing, and to find sheltered workshop placement.

Transition Planning

When the Treatment Team accepts the resident's Pre-release/Aftercare application, a general plan for full transition is outlined. Preparing residents for community living and preventing further sexual offenses are major goals of the plan. A transition checklist (see Appendix Q) is placed in the resident's chart. To formalize this new focus, the CTT reviews the plan

---

[2] Even though they may not be in full agreement, staff support the client's Aftercare plan and help him accomplish it as an exercise in making decisions and taking responsibility for their consequences.

with the resident and helps prepare him emotionally for the change. At this time, all major Inhouse treatment is being completed and he is given an MMPI.[3]

Pre-release/Aftercare Groups

Clients within a few months of transition may attend some Inhouse groups and activities while beginning Pre-release/Aftercare groups. The closer the client is to Aftercare, the more outside (off-unit) activities he attends. Initially, off-unit activities are done in a group with staff supervision. Later on, groups of two or more Aftercare clients participate in unsupervised off-unit activities together (e.g., going to a movie).

All clients attend four basic groups in the Pre-release/Aftercare component: relapse prevention, debriefing, support, and leisure groups. These groups reinforce training for community living by solidifying Inhouse learning, providing a safe and supportive environment for the client's "new me," monitoring the client's condition in the community, and providing feedback to improve the effectiveness of Inhouse treatment.

Relapse Prevention. The relapse prevention model (see Appendix R) was initially developed for substance abusers and was then adapted for use with sex offenders (Pithers, Marques, Gibat, & Marlatt, 1983).[4] The SSP has made several adaptations in the relapse prevention model to increase its effectiveness with lower functioning clients: simpler language, shorter sequencing requirements, more emphasis on coping response rehearsals ("what-to-do's"), and more attention to experiential learning.

Relapse is a sequential process occurring over time and involving the interaction of a number of risk factors. Relapse is predictable; therefore, early intervention makes relapse prevention possible. Some identified risk factors include affective, behavioral, cognitive, environmental, physiological, psychological, spiritual, interpersonal, and treatment issues (Daly, 1987). In the relapse prevention workshop these factors are called "set-ups."

"Set-ups" are divided into "set-up feelings," "set-up thinking," and "set-up situations." In Relapse Prevention sessions each resident identifies his personal "what-to-do's" and practices them in various situations. The participant also develops an emergency plan (placed on the back of his Crisis Card) to counter "slips" (lapses) without "giving up." "Slips" are

---

[3] An MMPI is also administered just before release and at six to nine months after release in order to monitor progress.

[4] For an overview of Relapse Prevention and specific adaptations for sex offenders, see also Laws (1989).

identified as fantasies, strong urges, or masturbation to aberrant themes. "Giving up" is when a client "slips" and then begins viewing himself as hopeless (abstinence violation effect). Without intervention, this frame of mind leads to relapse (reoffense).

The workshop is taught in 16 90-minute sessions. Each session has a specific objective that contributes to the goal of maintaining abstinence. Each class includes a short demonstration by staff and small group or individual projects prescriptively assigned to each resident. Below are examples of relapse prevention lesson plans.

Focus: Set-up thinking

Objective: The resident will be able to dispute three set-up thinking errors.

Methods:

Opening demonstration. Staff act out a role play of a resident asking his CTT for permission for his father to visit. The father has a similar crime history and has currently been charged with a new sex offense. Staff believe that the father represents a security risk for the client, and his visit is denied by the Treatment Team. Cartoon-type thought balloons are held up behind each actor's head to reveal how his self-talk might differ from what he is saying out loud.

Discussion. Staff ask, "What were the thinking errors? What appears to be okay? How could these thinking errors lead to reoffense?" Answers are listed on a flipchart.

Individual/small group projects. Every group member draws from a deck three cards, each of which has a specific sexually deviant thinking error on it. He tells the other residents in his small group what is wrong with each thinking error and then explains the correct thinking. He asks other residents for feedback. When he is successfully able to dispute three thinking errors in a row he is presented a "superior marksmanship" medal at a brief awards ceremony during lunch. Each resident continues practicing until he is successful.

Focus: Set-up feelings interventions

Objective: The residents will recognize that their feelings are not always an accurate reflection of the true situation.

Methods:

Opening Demonstration. An excerpt from the movie *Eye of the Beholder*[5] is shown. Staff lead a discussion about how various characters in the movie differed in their feelings about the main character based on their interactions with him.

Staff tell the story of "The Blind Men and the Elephant." Residents discuss how each blind man perceived the elephant based on touching the elephant in a different place from the others.

Individual/small group project. The class is divided into groups of three and directed to prepare a skit about how to intervene with their "set-up feelings" using the "1, 2, 3 method": (1) ask a safe friend to listen; (2) make "I feel ... because" statement; (3) listen to the friend's perception.

Homework. Each resident monitors his "set-up feelings" in a journal or a graph. He names the feeling and rates its intensity daily. When the intensity of the feeling reaches a certain level the client activates the "1, 2, 3 method."

Focus: Set-up situations

Objective: The resident will identify personal set-up situations.

Methods:

Opening Demonstration. Staff put sand in residents' shoes and direct them to walk around, asking how it feels. The staff add small stones, asking how it feels, then add larger stones and again ask how it feels. Staff discuss how big problems start with small signs that seem unimportant and if not dealt with early, lead to "big trouble."

Individual Project. Staff direct residents to make drawings, collages, or video scenarios of their personal "set-up situations." Each resident presents his project to the group and explains how he could avoid such situations or get out of them early.

By the end of the workshop clients have developed a Crisis Card to carry with them summarizing their set-ups, what-to-do's, and emergency plans. The last instruction on the card is "If I reoffend, I will turn myself in."[6]

---

[5] See Resources for film availability.

[6] One client actually turned himself in.

In a weekly Pre-release/Aftercare group they review set-ups they may have encountered during the week and how they coped.

Debriefing groups. Led by staff, these groups meet for 30 minutes, three times a week, during which time the client has an opportunity to discuss whatever is bothering him. The group gives him immediate feedback and helps him understand how he could have handled the situation differently. The positive and supportive group atmosphere encourages the client to apply his learning to the community setting.

Support group. This general group meets for two purposes: (1) to allow open discussion of such client issues as relapse cycles, difficulties with relationships, or other stressors encountered during the week; and (2) to discuss such logistical issues as client-planned trips, community passes, special permissions for unusual activities, and "accountabilities" for Pre-release clients still on the unit.

The group meetings may be held in the Aftercare Therapist's office or in an Aftercare client's apartment. When members meet in a client's home, they might cook together, building skills and group cohesiveness. Occasionally, ex-Aftercare clients attend meetings to receive and give encouragement.

Leisure group. This group is designed to provide the typical SSP client with appropriate community leisure experiences, an essential element in transition planning. Facilitated by the Recreational Therapist, the group, mostly sex offenders, spends one week planning safe community activities and the next week implementing them. Inexpensive or free activities accessible to clients after they have left the SSP include movies at a local community college, dress rehearsals for local plays, community adult volleyball, eating out, and parties at a client's home. After each outing clients discuss their feelings, thoughts, and behaviors.

The resident continues to work in these four group settings, focusing on his primary treatment issue with special attention to its relationship to his survival in the community. At the same time he is fully involved and accountable to his inpatient group and Therapy Supervisor. Because the resident experiences role confusion during this tense period, his inpatient identity must be maintained and supported while preparing him for Pre-release.

Transition Process

Six months prior to release, the resident begins to experience the full impact of "separation." He begins a half-time, off-unit hospital work assignment and goes on community outings with peers. During this rapid transition period the resident is supported by his CTT who continues to work with him on a one-to-one basis, writing and monitoring his treatment plan until just prior to release. Accountability and supervision then shift to the Transition Therapy Supervisor, with whom the resident works to build rapport while becoming acquainted with the Aftercare support staff.

With staff help, the resident establishes a weekly schedule to monitor and coordinate his activities, maintain structure, and train himself in time management. Initially, his weekly schedule includes a 20-hour, on-grounds hospital job and 20 hours of other transition-treatment activities.[7] Staff review, initial, and post the client's schedule in the staff office; copies may be given to the client's prospective group home or to structured alternative living staff. The resident keeps a copy of his schedule and is accountable for following it.

Four days a week, all Pre-release/Aftercare clients check in with each other and staff to review the day's victories and defeats, to coordinate activities schedules, to deal with out-of-control behavior, and to keep a treatment focus through transition.

Redefining the Client's Relationship to the Unit

As the resident nears release, his relationship to the unit, the staff, and the other residents intentionally changes. He is encouraged to think of the unit as a long-term "home base" where he sees himself more as a volunteer or auxiliary staff than as a resident. Staff not directly involved in the treatment plan take a friendly and supportive stance toward the Pre-release resident much as they would toward a student or volunteer.

Parole Planning

During the months prior to parole, the Treatment Team meets to approve the resident's discharge plan and draw up a discharge contract (see Appendix C), treatment focus, and level of supervision. The Therapy Supervisor coordinates all the resources involved, including the parole board and parole officer, release services, and various community agencies and support systems. The Therapy Supervisor begins one-to-one counseling with the resident, building rapport to ensure that a stable structure is in place several months before parole, so that on the parole date only his address changes. The CTT becomes a consultant to the transition staff and a resource person for the resident should he become anxious about the changes taking place in his life.

---

[7] Both Pre-release and Aftercare clients plan and carry out two to four hours of high visibility unit volunteer time in their weekly schedules.

Early Discharge (0-6 months)

In order to maintain consistency of treatment, the client returns to the unit daily through the week and at least once on the weekend to check in, volunteer time, or just socialize. All Pre-release programming continues and is monitored on the resident's weekly schedule, on which he also accounts for any unstructured time. He is encouraged to spend his leisure time with peers.

An automatic condition of parole in many jurisdictions is not to associate with other ex-cons. Since peer support is crucial to the success of the program, the SSP by design involves parole officers in every phase of the Pre-release/Aftercare program; association with other SSP peers is encouraged, not restricted.

The client lives either in sheltered housing or with an SSP peer. He is encouraged to seek peer help in finding community support systems and adjusting to being outside the institution. As he becomes emotionally attached in the community, he is urged to shift from the SSP's support systems to those of the community.

To facilitate and monitor his progress, the transition staff actively seek contact with the resident's family, employer, close friends, pastors, or others. As needed, the Aftercare Skills Trainer meets with residents on the unit or in clients' homes to conduct informal training in living skills: basic nutritional needs (food preparation and cooking); sex and dating; health care; apartment maintenance/emergencies; and community resources. Every Aftercare client is offered one-to-one counseling on a regular basis, either to monitor progress or to concentrate on particular issues that emerge. In addition, couples counseling is offered when necessary.

Aftercare clients receive continuing alcohol/drug treatment, which helps them in adjusting to and attending AA and NA meetings, getting a sponsor, and socializing with others within the recovering community. Because they feel safe there, Aftercare clients initially attend the Correctional Treatment Programs' AA meetings, where they model for inpatient clients how to be involved. If Antabuse[8] is ordered by the Treatment Team, its use is monitored by the unit staff; periodic urinalyses are provided as needed.

---

[8] *Antabuse* (disulfiram) prevents the normal breakdown of alcohol in the body, causing a toxic reaction. A person on Antabuse who drinks alcohol may experience effects ranging from nausea and vomiting to, in extreme cases, convulsions and cardiac arrhythmia (Barnhart, 1988, p. 637).

In Aftercare the client continues to work on sexual deviancy issues with his inpatient BT, in one-to-one counseling with the Aftercare Therapy Supervisor, and in group. Attendance at on-unit and off-unit SA[9] meetings is encouraged. His progress is monitored with sexual re-assessments completed prior to release, six months into Aftercare (if there are indications of regression), and before discharge.

To ensure effective use of his vocational skills and to encourage his financial independence whenever possible, the Aftercare client is provided appropriate vocational skills training. Beginning with his on-grounds hospital work site, the focus is on client contact with employees and staff support. While he is re-adjusting to the work environment, the client is closely monitored by staff to help him work through any problems with co-workers or supervisors. In conducting a job search, the SSP works with the Aftercare client and outside agencies, while carefully maintaining a balance between the client's need for support and the demands of the job search. When community or sheltered employment is secured, the SSP works with the employer and the Aftercare client to improve communication and to work out any problems.

Later Post-release (6-12 months)

Though support programming continues while the Aftercare client adjusts to community living, he is less accountable to the SSP for his time and budget. Staff are less actively involved with his support people, working toward an eventual "crisis-support" role. He undergoes a new arousal assessment and MMPI, and while still under supervision, his trial period use of Antabuse is reviewed. By now the client has a solid social and treatment support network in the community to help him become more self-sufficient.

Graduation

When the client completes all phases of the program and is prepared to move into the community as a fully independent "new me," a formal ceremony is held including all those who have been important in his metamorphosis: correctional staff, community support people, consultants, and so forth. At the graduation party, the client's friends and guests celebrate his progress, congratulate him on his success, and share refreshments prepared by unit residents.

---

[9] Sexaholics Anonymous (SA) focuses on sexual addiction in a 12-step program similar to that of AA.

CASE STUDY

Steve

OFFENSE HISTORY

Presenting Offense

Steve agreed to treatment in the SSP after being convicted and incarcerated for second degree burglary.

Prior Offenses

Steve had been previously arrested for a variety of offenses: possession of drugs, burglaries, larcenies, trespassing, shoplifting, and attempted rapes. He spent a total of six years in prison for these offenses. The records show that Steve did not respond to attempts at supervision while on probation or parole. While living in the community, he made threats and assaults when the authorities tried to apprehend him.

BACKGROUND INFORMATION

Steve is a 37-year-old white male (age 30 at SSP admission) with an extremely troubled background. Short and stocky, with a large head, close-set eyes, and a speech impediment, he was often mistaken for a more severely disabled person. His explosive temper had an intensely negative impact on his social life.

Steve was the second of five children and was raised in small towns and rural areas. His parents were abusive and Steve's memories of his homelife were terrifying. He often told the story of how his parents tried to "feed him to the pigs" on the family farm. Once his mother tried to drown him in the bathtub. He recalled that when he acted out as a child, he would be "locked in the basement for days" at a time.

Child protection authorities removed Steve from his home at age 13. He was placed in and ran away from four different foster homes, later returning to burglarize each of them, ransacking the house and stealing food. Steve's explosive temper (typically expressed by yelling abusive language at ear-splitting volume and throwing things) made it difficult for him to fit in anywhere.

By age 14, Steve was clearly out of control and had been involved in burglary, assault, and firesetting incidents. He was sentenced to reform school for one year. He escaped 15 times. He continued to exhibit aggressive and explosive behaviors toward both peers and staff.

After his release from reform school, his troubling behavior continued. According to his self-report, he became involved in a Satanic cult in another state, where he stole goods that the group's members sold to finance drug purchases. One day he and a friend simply left, returning to Oregon in search of Steve's family, who had moved away without telling him. In the next decade, he was constantly in trouble and arrested for burglaries, larcenies, drug possession, trespassing, shoplifting, and attempted rapes.

He was first admitted to a mental institution at age 20 with a diagnosis of paranoid schizophrenia. The records show that Steve was unsupervisable on probation/parole. When the authorities tried to apprehend him for his offenses, he made threats, committed assaults, and made several suicide attempts. He was readmitted to hospitals annually until his third and last incarceration in prison at age 28, for burglary. His behavior was so disruptive that he eventually was placed in the psychiatric security unit for his own protection and then referred to the SSP. At the screening interview Steve was hallucinating and very agitated. He denied that he had any major problems, but reluctantly stated a willingness to try treatment in the SSP.

Work History

According to all available sources, Steve had never held any kind of job, volunteer or paid, before entering the SSP.

TREATMENT REVIEW

Orientation

When Steve first came into the program, he tried his abusive, tough guy approach with staff and residents. The residents were scared of him and staff were apprehensive around him.

Clinical Assessment

Steve's clinical assessment produced a complex picture of an individual with multiple problems and few adaptive skills. Based on the *DSM III-R* Steve was diagnosed as follows:

Axis I: Paranoid Schizophrenic
Organic Mental Syndrome
Substance Abuse

Axis II: Borderline Personality Disorder with antisocial and dependent features
Borderline Intellectual Functioning (WAIS-R full scale IQ: 70)

Axis III: Obesity
Speech Impediment

Steve's central dynamic seemed to be his rage at rejection, a feature of Borderline Personality Disorder. Besides the drawbacks of his unattractive physical appearance and poor social skills, Steve was depressed as a result of his agitated sense of abandonment. He exhibited many self-defeating behaviors and had episodes of intermittent explosiveness. Steve displayed a sense of generalized rage in his assaultiveness, rape attempts, and firesetting. But despite all these deficits, he had developed at least one effective coping skill: he could charm and involve staff in enabling ways.

During Orientation, the SSP psychiatrist reviewed the medications that Steve had taken in prison and decided to reduce their level. The psychiatrist met with Steve on an ongoing basis to monitor his hallucinations.

Containment of Negative Behaviors

When Steve came into the SSP, the first general intervention focused on containing his explosive behaviors. He was placed in the Phoenix family and provided a clear structure with firm limits and a high level of staff attention. His initial response to the new experience and to limit-setting was positive. The containment strategy paired Steve with a "high status" buddy on the unit. He then became involved in the basic living skills modules and was compliant in that setting.

Steve attended the workshops and groups in the areas of sexual deviancy and alcohol/drug treatment. The primary treatment plan, however, continued to focus on containment of his explosiveness through the development of an anger management behavior contract, specifying that Steve would be debriefed by staff twice a day and would acquire skills for handling anger situations. His first step was to learn how to walk away from difficult situations and take a voluntary break from the activity. At this point a cognitive *Stop* statement was introduced, but had little impact. His second step was rehearsing anger management skills in role plays that were videotaped, giving Steve visual, auditory, and behavioral feedback on how he behaved in such situations.

Inhouse Treatment

During his first six months on the unit there were two distinct stages: a "honeymoon" period which lasted about three months, followed by three months of testing the program limits.

In one of his first rounds of limit-testing Steve stopped taking his medication and became verbally aggressive with everyone. His yells literally shook the building with jolts that could be heard on the other units.

A major feature of Steve's borderline personality was his polarized, black/white thinking. When residents and staff did what Steve wanted, they were "good," and Steve felt good. When they did not do what he wanted, they were "bad," and Steve became physically aggressive. His issues became more predominant when staff unwittingly reinforced this "splitting process" by attending to the "Angel Steve" and neglecting the task of developing the "Gray

Steve," a person who (like everyone else) does good, bad, and in-between things. Staff began to relax the limits and structure that had been originally set for him, eroding the consistency of limit-setting. He eventually became so abusive and explosive that he was returned to the prison for two weeks in order to regain his attention before readmitting him to the SSP.

His pattern of abusiveness and assaultiveness continued over the length of his treatment. *Steve was returned to the prison and readmitted seven times.* Every return to prison involved his fear of abandonment, and it became clear that this fear was a key to his acting out on the unit as well as a central dynamic in his criminal behavior in the community.

Steve's risk factors for reoffending were identified as his acting out, organic impairments, alcohol/drug abuse, mental illness, and his poor impulse control, which expressed itself in explosiveness. Treatment interventions addressed his personality disorder, medical/psychiatric needs, alcohol/drug issues, sexual deviancy patterns, and transition competencies.

Personality Disorder

In addressing Steve's personality disorder, the central focus was on anger management. Steve had to learn to accept his own limitations, which became the "new button" that he developed in the anger management workshop. He also was given help in dealing with his cognitive distortions around his "black or white, good or bad" thinking. The idea that there are "gray" areas in people was emphasized. His *Stop* statement was, "It's not worth it"; his *Go* statement was, "I can make it." From his many years of yelling, he was able to proclaim these statements with great gusto.

Steve was assigned a three-part journal focus: (1) to identify two times a day how people were pushing him away; (2) to relate how he used smart self-talk to deal with the rejection; and (3) to explain how he checked out his view of the situation.

One attempt at dealing with his abandonment issues was to provide him with grief counseling around the loss of his family. He had had no contact with them for 10 years and had heard that they were all dead.

Medical/Psychiatric

In the course of his treatment Steve had periods of regression, during which he hallucinated and had suicidal ideations. These problems were generally precipitated by his "cheeking" his medications or deliberately vomiting them.

The SSP's general treatment approach was to educate him to the role that medication played in his mental health: it empowered his "new me" behaviors. Through this empowering process he eventually was able to maintain himself successfully on his medication on the unit.

The issue of obesity was addressed through education on diet and nutrition and building an image of his "new me." He charted his own weight loss as a measurement of his success. He was doing very well with his weight loss until Thanksgiving, when his Therapy Supervisor suggested that since he had been doing so well, a "vacation" from his diet would be okay. Steve ate steadily for three days and regained all the weight he had lost.[1] However, after release from the SSP Steve lost weight.

Alcohol/Drug Abuse

Steve attended the SSP's six alcohol and drug modules and the unit AA meetings. Steve's treatment plan involved education regarding the effects of alcohol and drugs on his maintenance medications. Although he was willing to be involved, Steve maintained denial of his substance abuse problem while in the Inhouse phase of treatment and never demonstrated a high commitment to abstinence.

Sexual Deviancy

Steve cooperated in giving a psychosexual history and consented to an arousal assessment involving the penile plethysmograph. This combination helped develop a clinical picture to determine the course of treatment for his sexually deviant behaviors.

---

[1] The SSP has since discontinued focusing on obesity—most clients lose some weight when they leave the institutional setting because they are more active and eat less food.

Steve's psychosexual history revealed that he had very limited sexual experience. He was preoccupied with adult women and seemed to have an unquenchable need for affection and acceptance. His lack of social skills, combined with his "odd" looks, general aggressiveness, emotional volatility, and unrealistic judgments as to who would make a suitable mate, limited his ability to develop a satisfactory relationship.

He reported that the two attempted rapes took place during periods of extreme loneliness and that in each case the victims had been friendly but had rejected his advances. One was a stranger, the other his sister's friend for whom he had bought a beer. When he was rebuffed in both cases he attempted to force the women to have sex. He stated that at the time he thought they were "just trying to play a game" with him.

During his plethysmograph evaluation Steve showed high arousal to female adult mutual scenes and moderate arousal to rape themes, then lost tumescence as the taped scenarios became exclusively violent. He had low arousal to female child slides and tapes and no arousal to assault scenarios, adult males, or male children. He was able to distinguish between ages very accurately. This physiological assessment matched his self-reported sexual history.

It appeared that his sexual acting out was not driven by rape fantasies, but was apparently another manifestation of his rage over being rejected, poor coping skills, and resulting frustration.

Several goals specific to sexual deviancy were identified: (1) reducing and controlling Steve's rape urges by using covert sensitization to learn and rehearse the consequences to himself and the victim if he were to act out again; (2) desensitizing him to nonsexual interactions with female adults; and (3) improving his social image by teaching hygiene, proper attire, appropriate social distance, and good personal grooming. Other important steps for Steve to avoid reoffending were continuing to take his medications, abstaining from street drugs and alcohol, and structuring his time.

To treat his sexually deviant urges, first Steve was assigned to watch video tapes of rape victims telling how they suffered as a result of being abused. He took notes and included that information in his covert sensitization audio tapes when he focused on consequences to his victims. Initially he was resistive and at times belligerent over this assignment. Staff walked Steve through the victim empathy process several times, apparently because he did not understand the assignment and was unwilling to "look dumb" by asking for help. With increased individual help and repetition, he began catching on. He intuitively had a better understanding of victim perspectives than many higher functioning clients. He developed great pride in his skill in making covert sensitization tapes and demonstrated his ability to control his deviant urges in the behavioral therapy lab during assessments. Some of his tapes were used for training higher functioning clients on other sex-offender units, and eventually he became a tutor for other SSP residents. After 12 weeks of daily tapes he went to a maintenance schedule of two audio tapes weekly. He credited this treatment as having the greatest impact on his becoming a "new me."

To desensitize him in nonsexual interactions with adult women, Steve was assigned to work on assertiveness training with a female psychology intern.[2] To avoid Steve's abandonment issues, it was clearly defined at the outset how long the sessions would run. Gradually, as he participated in a number of assertiveness training exercises with the intern, he appeared to gain confidence and some competence. During the third week Steve became upset and pouted when he observed the intern talking to another resident. She again clarified her role both on the unit and with him specifically; this explanation seemed to improve his mood. At the end of the 12 weeks Steve appeared to be very comfortable with the intern, and more at ease in general around women staff members on the unit.

Next, Steve began a second round of weekly assertiveness training sessions with a female staff member to help him work on

[2] It has been the SSP's experience that telling clients they were going to learn to be more comfortable with women often has the opposite effect. The assignments are therefore somewhat disguised.

his interactions. Steve improved his skills by taping role plays of various situations and assertive responses and then reviewing the video tapes in debriefing sessions.

He worked on creating a new social image by making a collage with pictures cut from magazines depicting his "old self" and his "new self." He also had a peer rate him on his appearance daily and self-charted the result. Overall he improved his appearance and his attention to social cues. When he felt abandoned his attention to his appearance waned, but it again improved as his mood improved.

Transitional Competencies

Steve developed basic living skills by attending classes in personal grooming and basics, telephone usage, sex education, and other basic training modules. He was involved in activity therapies, but due to poor coordination and aggressiveness, he often injured himself and others. The Treatment Team thus decided to involve him in more passive activities; he did well in ceramics, specializing in "one-eyed" turtles.

Transition and Aftercare

During the Pre-release phase of his treatment, Steve was expected to take a greater responsibility for setting his own limits, an extremely difficult task for him. The closer his release date came and the more his limits were loosened, the greater his fears of abandonment grew. As expected, Steve had great difficulty handling the ambiguity of the transition phase. To counter the problem, staff devised a special technique: the "ice cream intervention." The Therapy Supervisor (TS) and the Aftercare Therapist (ACT) "fought" for Steve's attention. The ACT would argue within Steve's earshot in favor of taking Steve out on a pass for ice cream. The TS would feign resistance, establishing a sense of security for Steve. Steve saw the ACT as a person who really wanted a caring relationship. Of course, the ACT "won" these "arguments" and the two left the unit for ice cream. This scenario was played out for several months while the therapeutic alliance between the ACT and Steve developed. Meanwhile, the TS expressed an active interest in how Steve was doing and provided input on his treatment.

Steve's Aftercare plan included working with the county MR/DD agency to find housing. He eventually was placed at a group home for mentally ill clients. The move was accomplished in stages. First, to give him the opportunity to meet the other residents and to ask questions, Steve visited the group home for several brief periods with SSP staff. In the second stage, he spent some time on his own at the home and ate a meal there. In the third stage Steve was given a day-long pass at the home, and in the fourth stage he was issued an overnight pass to get a feeling for what it was like to be off the unit for an extended period of time. Steve was fully debriefed by the ACT and his Pre-release/Aftercare support group. In the fifth stage Steve was placed on temporary leave for six months, so that when things got out of control, he could be returned to the SSP as a crisis intervention.

This transition to community living was quite rocky, and relationships with the other residents and staff of the group home and the SSP were sometimes volatile. The group home staff had the option to call the SSP and request Steve's immediate return when he became uncontrollable, an option they exercised three times. However, each time Steve went through this process he made some progress. By the time Steve's parole release was mandatory, he had settled in fairly well to group home living. His leisure activities tended toward going out for coffee or to a budget movie with other Aftercare clients or group home residents.

Steve had his own room and TV at the group home and took considerable pride in being able to live semi-independently. However, during his Aftercare period of supervision there were a number of crises. He tested the limits to see if the SSP still cared by smoking marijuana, which counteracted the effectiveness of his medications. Eventually, he weathered this crisis by accepting more realistically his need for the medication and realizing how badly affected he was by mixing street drugs with it.

Steve continued treatment by coming back to the unit to attend Aftercare treatment groups and sexual deviancy treatment. He also became involved with a rehabilitation training program, where he learned to grade and stack lumber for pallets, earning a percentage of the competitive wage based on his productivity.

While his experience at that program was stormy at first, he was again supported through the adjustment by the SSP and the group home staff. With the SSP taking the lead in directing the general flow of treatment, the group home, the SSP, and the rehabilitation training program formed a coordinated, cooperative network to share information, provide structure and monitor his schedule, and set limits for Steve. The ACT met weekly with Steve at the group home and at the rehabilitation program.

During the course of his Aftercare Steve discovered information that created emotional upheaval in his life: his supposedly dead parents were in fact living about 16 miles from his group home. When he contacted them by phone, they seemed interested in seeing him and arrangements were made for him to visit them with the ACT. The first visit was very stiff and uncomfortable for everyone. Steve's parents gave no explanation for their lack of contact and Steve was afraid to ask.

Steve was frequently debriefed around the rediscovery of his family. His retarded older sister seemed to be the only member of his family who genuinely responded to him, and his relationship with her became a significant one. But about four months after the reunion, Steve's sister suddenly died and he experienced a huge sense of loss. During his renewed grief counseling, Steve went to his sister's grave and told her that she was the only family member who understood him and that he loved her.

Soon after his sister's death, Steve's family once again moved without telling him their whereabouts. Though this was a blow to him, Steve seemed more able to accept the loss. The SSP and the group home provided crucial support at this time.

Steve also had a health crisis soon after his sister's death: he contracted Guillain-Barre Syndrome and was fully paralyzed for almost three months. He was placed in a nursing home for another two months of recovery. By the time he was ready to return to the community he was off parole and formal Aftercare supervision had ended. A new co-ed group home was located about 16 miles from the SSP.

The SSP continued to work with him on a reduced basis. Steve seemed to be able to handle the stress of the move fairly well, and although his physical problems slowed him down somewhat, he took more seriously his need for medical intervention.

The ACT's biweekly visits soon were changed to monthly contacts. After a year Steve moved to a satellite apartment but continued to spend a lot of time at the co-ed group home. He had begun taking great interest in a woman resident who had some deficits he could help her with. They started living together, and about a year later were married.

Steve continues to have mental health problems. Twice he became too optimistic about how things were going and discontinued taking his medication. Both times he decompensated, had suicidal ideations, and spent two brief periods in the state hospital until he was again stabilized on medications. ***He has remained in the community crime-free for six years.***

7

OUTCOMES: BREAKING NEW GROUND

Compared to nondisabled sex offenders, intellectually disabled sex offenders are not a large population in numbers. But like their nondisabled counterparts, they have a large and painful impact on the community. In 1987, data collected for an inhouse study on the 17 sex offenders who were then in the SSP revealed that they had committed 3300 separate sex offenses against 250 victims.

The pain of victims, of the community, and of the offender will not be reduced until society recognizes and deals with the problem of sexual abuse proactively. Effective treatment for intellectually disabled sex offenders holds part of the answer of how to begin decreasing community pain by reducing the incidence of sexual crimes. The authors of this book feel increasingly confident and optimistic that quality treatment programming benefits the offender, the various systems involved with the offender, and the community at large.

Measuring "Success"

Specialized treatment for intellectually disabled sex offenders is a relatively new field; in a very real sense, clinicians in the SSP and elsewhere are breaking new ground. Because there are no longitudinal outcome data for other programs treating intellectually disabled sex offenders, there is currently no adequate way to establish the SSP's relative "success" or "failure." Comparisons with outcome data from treatment programs for nondisabled sex offenders are equally inadequate, since such studies for this population are also lacking.

The SSP's outcome data fall into two categories, "objective" and "subjective." The "objective" data consist of a study of post-treatment recidivism rates of SSP clients. A growing body of analysis (Furby, Weinrott, & Blackshaw, 1989; Tracy, Donnelly, Morgenbesser, & Macdonald, 1983) casts doubt on the relevance, usefulness, and accuracy of recidivism studies as a measure of treatment success. Recidivism rates do not give a complete picture of the impact treatment might have on reducing the number of victims or the severity of assaultive behavior. Nor do recidivism rates take into consideration the gross underreportage of sexual crimes, currently estimated at no more than 10 percent of actual occurrences (Furby et al., 1989, p. 27). Further, as Quinsey and Marshall (1983) note, "Recidivism presents a problem as a measure of treatment success since it reflects not only repeated offending, but also police efficiency, the offender's luck or improved criminal skills, and a variety of other factors beyond experimental control" (p. 269). But because the question, "What is your recidivism rate?" is always asked, data on SSP clients are provided.

The real questions, of course, are, "Does your program work?" and "How do you know that it works?" In an attempt to answer those questions, the SSP also considers such "subjective" data as case studies and increases in skills and functioning levels.[1]

Both objective and subjective data are influenced by the length of time clients stay in treatment. Approximately 20 percent of the residents are terminated from the SSP because of assaultive behavior or serious rule infractions; 25 percent voluntarily terminate their treatment. Of these, approximately 35 percent return to the parent institution because of lack of motivation. Of the unmotivated 35 percent, approximately 33 percent are readmitted to the SSP after a brief stay in the parent institution. Clients' overall length of stay in the program varies: approximately 15 percent of the residents return to the parent institution after two months; 40 percent return after two to twelve months; and 45 percent complete more than 12 months of treatment.

While admittedly problematic from a research scientist's point of view, both objective and subjective categories of data indicate that treatment for the intellectually disabled sex offender decreases the client's tendency to reoffend.

Objective Data: Recidivism

The SSP's objective data indicate that treatment decreases the criminal activity of program participants. In 1989 the SSP conducted an outcome study examining the post-treatment criminal activity of residents admitted to the SSP from 1979 to 1988 (N=199) using the Law Enforcement Data Systems (LEDS) for recidivism reports.[2] *Recidivism* was conservatively defined as "any felony crime conviction" (which could include

---

[1] Defining and developing clearer and more precise objective measurement tools and evaluating each of the many treatment areas is a priority for SSP staff.

[2] The study initially examined the records of all 268 clients who had been admitted to the SSP from 1979 to 1988. Because no LEDS data were available for 69 clients in two groups (those who had left the state and those who had been returned to prison after treatment and remained there), they were excluded.

driving on a suspended license, trespassing, criminal misconduct, and fourth degree assault). The results of the study are summarized in Table 1.

Table 1

Recidivism Rates of All Residents
(Sex Offenders and Non-sex Offenders)
By Length of Time in SSP Treatment and Community Aftercare Services, 1979-88

	Length of Time in Treatment	Recidivism Rate
(N=57)	90 days or less	65%
(N=36)	90 to 180 days	78%
(N=29)	181 to 365 days	65%
(N=28)	366 to 545 days	50%
(N=49)	greater than 545 days	39%
(N=35)	with Aftercare services	29%

These data indicate that the longer the client is involved in treatment (one year or more), the less likely he is to reoffend. The most dramatic drop in recidivism occurs when clients receive community Aftercare services.

In examining the relapses of *sex offenders* from 1979 through 1988 (see Table 2), a different, *offense-specific* definition of recidivism was used: "committing a new *sexual* offense." Under this new definition, the recidivism rate for sex offenders (N=62)[3] was 23 percent, compared to a recidivism rate under the old definition (including all types of offenses) of 44 percent.

Table 2

Recidivism Rates of Sex Offenders by Length of Time in the SSP, 1979-1988

	Length of Time in Treatment	Recidivism Rate All crimes	Recidivism Rate Sexual crimes
(N=28)	365 days or less	54%	25%
(N=34)	greater than 365 days	35%	21%
(N=62)	overall	44%	23%

[3] This number includes 11 sex offenders admitted between 1979 and 1982 who did not receive sex-offender-specific treatment programming.

Although all criminal activity within this population was not eliminated, these data clearly indicate that (1) specialized treatment had an impact on the criminal activity of these sex offenders in the SSP; and (2) clients in treatment for longer periods of time received greater benefit, shown by their lower recidivism rate.

Subjective Data

A more subjective collection of data paints an encouraging portrait of the SSP's effect on its clients:

• In the past 10 years, over 80 percent of offenders admitted to the SSP completed the Orientation phase of treatment and they:

— demonstrated competence in the basic living and treatment skills outlined in chapter 4;

— understood that thinking affects behavior; and

— identified their primary thinking error as well as other errors they have used throughout their lives.

• Over 50 percent of all offenders admitted to the SSP:

— developed and demonstrated competence in awareness of their drug or alcohol problem and their ability to function in an AA meeting;

— were able to use at least one treatment technique to reduce their arousal (measured by the penile plethysmograph);

— showed competence in basic living skills workshops;

— displayed their ability to manage anger outbursts; and

— established their ability to socialize and develop supportive interpersonal relationships.

• Offenders who were in the program for six months or more (50%) demonstrated an increase in their basic living skills and overall functioning level.

Benefits of Treatment to the Wider Community

In addition to the benefit of treatment to individual clients and the community in reducing the clients' tendency to reoffend, the SSP and similar programs have the potential to lessen community pain in a cost-effective manner. Some of the benefits to the wider community include:

• *Clinical knowledge increases.* Until recently, little was known about the potential for intellectually disabled offenders to control their behaviors. Through assessment and treatment, clinicians have begun to learn more about offender typologies, expand their understanding of offender patterns, and improve their ability to intervene more effectively and in a more timely manner.

• *Correctional and service systems become aware that intellectually disabled sex offenders have treatment options.* The SSP has been successful in providing quality treatment options for its sex-offender clients within the correctional system, increasing the awareness of correctional staff, other agencies, and community groups working with this population. The intellectually disabled offender now need not be so "lost" in the prison system: his higher profile means that he is more quickly identified, moved through the system, and appropriately referred for assistance with his behavioral problems.

• *The skills of correctional and other agencies increase.* Correctional staff, mental health agencies, group homes, probation/parole officers, judges, and individual treatment providers have benefited from learning the SSP's behavior-management techniques and treatment resources that can be used with this population in prison and upon their return to the community.

• *Intellectually disabled sex offenders become aware of their ability to manage their own problems and lives.* Because the SSP teaches its clients to survive in the community, they manage their lives better, utilize community services more effectively, and can stay in the community longer without offending. But despite the intellectually disabled sex offender's increased social skills and new ability to intervene in his aggressive behavior (as with all treated sex offenders), he may still choose to reoffend due to circumstances over which no treatment program has control.

A Testimonial

Testimonials are not scientific research, but they illustrate the kind of effect the SSP has on clients and the community and validate the program's design and direction. Examples like the one that follows suggest the SSP is on the right track, that treatment does make an impact:

> One 33-year-old client had never been in the community longer than three months since he was nine years old; he had always been in supervised settings. Every time he was released, he committed a crime, including over 12 rapes of different victims. His diagnosis included paranoid schizophrenia, mild mental retardation, and a very serious poly-drug problem. He was in the

SSP for a rather turbulent three years. As of 1989, he has been in the community for three and a half years. He maintains a consistent relationship with a womanfriend, has a good job, and visits the SSP often.

Elements of Quality Treatment Programs

Sex offenders, whether disabled or nondisabled, develop their maladaptive sexual behaviors over a long period of time. The behaviors do not go away with casual treatment for a few months. This serious, complex problem calls for quality treatment involving a major commitment of time and energy. A *quality* inpatient, long-term sex-offender treatment program combines organizational and clinical elements to create a supportive working and treatment environment.

Organizational Elements

Long before a single client is treated, an organizational structure must be in place that supports staff in accomplishing clinical goals. The following seven organizational elements are crucial to establishing a quality treatment program similar to the SSP:

• *The program must be a cooperative venture among all the agencies that deal with this population*: mental health, developmental disabilities, corrections departments (especially the parole board), and advocates for the civil rights and liberties of intellectually disabled clients. Mental health agencies contribute their expertise in changing behavior; corrections ensures public safety; developmental disabilities agencies specialize in caring for the intellectually disabled; and advocates monitor the process to prevent abuses.

• *All agencies involved must recognize that such a program takes leadership, and leaders may not make good administrators.* Leadership means taking risks; and as many administrators will confirm, there is little incentive and no reinforcement for risk-taking among state bureaucracies.

• *The program must create customized organizational systems which accommodate the treatment models.* Treatment must be a priority; trying to impose a radical new treatment system over an old administrative system fails both.

• *The program must include community training and the role of resource center.* From the beginning, the treatment program must educate the community and share its problems and successes in treating this population.

• *Staff training and supervision must be built in from the beginning.* There can be no quality treatment without ongoing staff training and good supervision.

• *Data collection systems must be incorporated from the start.* Data are the only indicators staff have to know whether the program is going in the right direction.

• *Program location requires careful attention.* The ideal location is off prison grounds in order for the clients to make a complete break from the convict culture of "us" against "them." A state psychiatric hospital location has advantages in providing security and access to the neuropsychiatric services this population may need and to other mental health professionals.

Clinical Elements

Quality treatment for intellectually disabled sex offenders is based on the following five clinical elements:

• *The program should be as voluntary as possible.* Being voluntary engages the client in his first step toward change as he says, "I want to be different."

• *The program must incorporate a multidiagnostic, holistic approach.* There is no room in this field for tunnel vision or narrow specialization by theoretical discipline. The client must be considered as a whole person; his treatment must be tailored to fit the way *all* of his abilities, disabilities, and history influence his behaviors and thoughts.

• *The program should be based on a self-help model* (e.g., modified therapeutic community). This model empowers the residents to participate in their own treatment and to create their own environment as much as possible. The environment is then used to reinforce the change process.

• *Cognitive restructuring, adapted to the kinds of reasoning problems the clients have* (e.g., using categorical learning and labeling, rather than inductive or deductive reasoning), *is a primary treatment tool.* It is used to address the clients' serious character disorders and distortions of thought and perception.

• *Learning should be fun.* Lessons are presented in "dramatic" or "bizarre" ways.

The SSP's staff and administrator hope other programs will follow its example, breaking new ground in treating intellectually disabled sex offenders, a severely underserved population. The creation of more quality programs across the country will dramatically increase the quality and availability of outcome data, which will in turn either validate the programs' effectiveness or contribute to reshaping the programs' treatment components, helping to create a safer society for us all.

REFERENCES

Abramson, P.R., Parker, T., & Weisberg, S.R. (1988). Sexual expression of mentally retarded people: Education and legal implications. *American Journal on Mental Retardation, 93*(3), 328-334.

American Psychiatric Association. (1987). *Diagnostic and statistical manual of mental disorders* (3rd ed., rev.). Washington, DC: Author.

Barnard, G.W., Fuller, A.K., Robbins, L., & Shaw, T. (1989). *The child molester: An integrated approach to evaluation and treatment.* New York: Brunner/Mazel.

Barnhart, E.R. (1988). *Physicians' Desk Reference* (42nd ed.). Oradell, NJ: Medical Economics Company.

Biklen, D.P. (1989). Redefining schools. In D. Biklen, D.L. Ferguson, & A. Ford (Eds.), *Schooling and disability* (pp. 1-24). Chicago: National Society for the Study of Education.

Biklen, D.P., & Mlinarcik, S. (1978). Criminal justice. Reprinted from J. Wortis (Ed.), *Mental retardation and developmental disabilities* (Vol. 10), (pp. 172-195). New York: Brunner/Mazel.

Blumer, D. (1970, February). Hypersexual episodes in temporal lobe epilepsy. *American Journal of Psychiatry, 126,* 1099-1106.

Coleman, E.M., & Murphy, W.D. (1980). A survey of sexual attitudes and sex education programs among facilities for the mentally retarded. *Applied Research in Mental Retardation, 1,* 269-276.

Crossmaker, M. (1986). *Empowerment: A systems approach to preventing assaults against people with mental retardation and/or developmental disabilities.* Columbus, OH: The National Assault Prevention Center.

Daly, D. (1987). Relapse prevention with substance abusers: Clinical issues and myths. *Social Work, 32*(2), 138-139.

Fried, E.R. (1986, May). *A multimodal treatment of developmentally disabled sex offenders.* Paper presented to the Fourth National Conference on the Sexual Victimization of Children, New Orleans, LA.

Furby, L., Weinrott, M.R., & Blackshaw, L. (1989). Sex offender recidivism: A review. *Psychological Bulletin, 105,* 3-30.

Gafgen, J. (1988, October). Taped interview by F.H. Knopp.

Gardner, H. (1983). *Frames of mind: Theory of multiple intelligences.* New York: Basic Books.

Graber, B., Hartman, K., Coffman, J., Huey, C., & Goldy, C. (1982, January). Brain damage among mentally disordered sex offenders. *Journal of Forensic Sciences, 27*(1), 125-134.

Griffiths, D.M., Quinsey, V.L., & Hingsburger, D. (1989). *Changing inappropriate sexual behavior: A community-based approach for persons with developmental disabilities.* Baltimore: Paul H. Brookes.

Hall, R.L. (1989). Assessment and diagnosis. In G.W. Barnard, A.K. Fuller, L. Robbins, & T. Shaw, *The child molester: An integrated approach to evaluation and treatment* (pp. 48-71). New York: Brunner/Mazel.

Jones, M. (1953). *The therapeutic community.* New York: Basic Books.

Knopp, F.H. (1984). *Retraining adult sex offenders: Methods & models.* Orwell, VT: The Safer Society Press.

Knopp, F.H., & Lackey, L.B. (1987). *Sexual offenders identified as intellectually disabled: A summary of data from 40 treatment providers.* Orwell, VT: The Safer Society Press.

Knopp, F.H. & Stevenson, W.F. (1989). *A nationwide survey of juvenile & adult sex-offender treatment programs and models, 1988.* Orwell, VT: The Safer Society Press.

Koloday, R.C., Masters, W.H., & Johnson, V.E. (1979). *Textbook of sexual medicine.* Boston: Little, Brown.

Laws, D.R. (Ed.). (1989). *Relapse prevention with sex offenders.* New York: Guilford Press.

Laws, D.R. & Osbourn, C.A. (1983). How to build and operate a behavioral laboratory to evaluate and treat sexual deviance. In J.G. Greer & I.R. Stuart (Eds.), *The sexual aggressor: Current perspectives on treatment* (pp. 293-335). New York: Van Nostrand Reinhold.

Lund, C. (1989, October). *Some useful principles in the assessment, management, and treatment of maladaptive, deviant, and illegal sexual behavior in retarded persons.* Paper presented at the 8th Annual Research and Data Conference, Association for the Behavioral Treatment of Sex Abusers, Seattle, WA.

Meichenbaum, D. (1977). *Cognitive behavioral modification.* New York: Plenum Press.

Miller, B.L., Cummings, J.L., McIntyre, H., Ebers, G., & Grode, M. (1986). Hypersexuality or altered sexual preference following brain injury. *Journal of Neurology, Neurosurgery, and Psychiatry, 49,* 867-873.

Murphy, W.D. & Barbaree, H. (1987). *Assessments of sexual offenders by measures of erectile response: Psychometric properties and decision making.* (Contract No. 86M0500501D). Washington, DC: National Institute of Mental Health.

Murphy, W.D., Coleman, E.M., & Haynes, M.R. (1983). Treatment and evaluation issues with the mentally retarded sex offender. In J.G. Greer & I.R. Stuart (Eds.), *The sexual aggressor: Current perspectives on treatment* (pp. 22-41). New York: Van Nostrand Reinhold.

Pithers, W.D., Kashima, K.M., Cumming, G.F., Beal, L.S., & Buell, M.M. (1988). Relapse prevention of sexual aggression. In R.A. Prentky & V.L. Quinsey (Eds.), *Human sexual aggression: Current perspectives* (p. 248). Annals of the New York Academy of Sciences Vol. 528. New York: The New York Academy of Sciences.

Pithers, W.D., Marques, J.K., Gibat, C.C., & Marlatt, G.A. (1983). Relapse prevention with sexual aggressives: A self-control model of treatment and maintenance of change. In J.G. Greer & I.R. Stuart (Eds.), *The sexual aggressor: Current perspectives on treatment* (pp. 214-239). New York: Van Nostrand Reinhold.

Quinsey, V.L. & Marshall, W.L. (1983). Procedures for reducing inappropriate sexual arousal: An evaluation review. In J.G. Greer & I.R. Stuart (Eds.), *The sexual aggressor: Current perspectives on treatment* (pp. 267-289). New York: Van Nostrand Reinhold.

Ross, R., Fabiano, E., & Earles, C. (1988). Reasoning and rehabilitation. *International Journal of Offender Therapy and Comparative Criminology, 32,* 30.

Safer Society Program (1988). *A summary of selected notes from the working sessions of the first national training conference on the assessment and treatment of intellectually disabled juvenile & adult sexual offenders, Columbus, Ohio, March 25-27, 1988.* The Working Sessions and The Training Conference on the Assessment and Treatment of Intellectually Disabled Juvenile & Adult Sexual Offenders was held under the auspices of the Ohio Youth Services Network (OYSN), The Safer Society Program, and other related Ohio agencies. The Working Sessions were attended by nine specialized treatment providers: Frank Caparulo, M.S., Center for Sexual Health and Education, Inc., CT; Michael Comte, M.S.W., A.C.S.W., Comte and Associates, WA; John Gafgen, B.A., Moderate Security Counseling & Treatment Unit, NJ; James Haaven, M.S., Social Skills Program, Oregon State Hospital, OR; Kathryn Kaufman, O.T.R., Sexual Disorders Clinic, Johns Hopkins Hospital, MD; Winifred Kempton, M.S.W., A.C.S.W., Private Consultant, PA; Laura Sissala, B.A., M.B.A., REM Lyndale, Inc., MN; J. Michael Whitaker, B.S., Youth Services Training Center, Allegheny Intensive Treatment Program, PA; and Ron Wilson, B.A., M.S., Sexuality Treatment & Training Program, Fairview Training Center, OR.

Salter, A.C. (1988). *Treating child sex offenders and victims: A practical guide.* Newbury Park, CA: Sage.

Santamour, M.B. (1986, Spring-Summer). The offender with mental retardation. *The Prison Journal, LXVI*(1) 3-18.

Santamour, M.B., & West, B. (1979). *Retardation and criminal justice—A training manual for criminal justice personnel.* Washington, DC: President's Committee on Mental Retardation.

Schwartz, M., & Masters, W. (1983). Conceptual factors in the treatment of paraphilias: A preliminary report. *Journal of Sex and Marital Therapy, 9,* 3-18.

Senn, C.Y. (1987). *Issues and questions involved in the sexual abuse of children with intellectual impairments.* Ontario, Canada: G. Allan Roeher Institute.

Sgroi, S.M. (1989). Evaluation and treatment of sexual offense behavior in persons with mental retardation. In S.M. Sgroi (Ed.), *Vulnerable populations* (Vol. 2, pp. 245-283). Lexington, MA: Lexington Books.

Steinhauser, C. (1989). *An analysis of covert sensitization and minimal arousal conditioning: A treatment outcome study.* Unpublished doctoral dissertation. University of Chicago.

Tracy, F., Donnelly, H., Morgenbesser, L., & Macdonald, D. (1983). Program evaluation: Recidivism research involving sex offenders. In J.G. Greer & I.R. Stuart (Eds.), *The sexual aggressor: Current perspectives on treatment* (pp. 198-213). New York: Van Nostrand Reinhold.

Weinstein, E.A. (1974, October). Sexual disturbances after brain injury. *Medical Aspects of Human Sexuality,* 10-31.

Willis, V. (1980, July). Design considerations for mental health facilities. *Hospital and Community Psychiatry, 31*(7) 483-490.

Yochelson, S. & Samenow, S. (1976-77). *Criminal personality* (Vols. 1-2). New York: J. Aronson.

Zilbergeld, B. (1978). *Male sexuality: A guide to sexual fulfillment.* Boston: Little, Brown.

RESOURCES

Films and Videos

Condom Sense. Available from Videograph, Perennial Education, Inc., 930 Pitner Avenue, Evanston, IL 60202. (1-800-323-9084)

Eye of the Beholder. Produced by General Electric (1953). Released by Stuart Reynolds Productions, distributed by BNA Communications, 9439 Key West Ave., Rockville, MD 20850. Phone 1-800-233-6067. This film may be available through your local public library.

Seventeen and Going Nowhere. Available from Paulist Productions, P.O. Box 1057, Pacific Palisades, CA 90272.

Soft is the Heart of a Child. Available from Hazelden Education Materials, Pleasant Valley Road, Box 176, Center City, MN 55012-0176.

Tests

Draw-A-Person (DAP). In Harris, D.B. (1963). *Children's drawings as measures of intellectual maturity.* New York: Harcourt Brace Jovanovich.

Halstead-Reitan battery. Available from Reitan Neuropsychology Laboratories, Inc., 1338 East Edison St., Tucson, AZ 85719.

Key Math Diagnostic Arithmetic Test, by A.J. Connelly, W. Nachtman, and E.M. Pritchett (1976). Available from American Guidance Service, Inc. Publishers' Building, Circle Pines, MN 55014.

Leisure Barriers Test. Unpublished manuscript, 1986. Peterson, C.A., Dunn, J.K., & Sneegas, J.J.

Millon Clinical Multiaxial Inventory, by Theodore Millon, Ph.D., (1976). Available from National Computer Systems, 4401 West 76th St. Minneapolis, MN 55435

Minnesota Multiphasic Personality Inventory, by R. Hathaway Starke, Ph.D., & J. Charnley McKinley, M.D. Available from Interpretive Scoring Systems, P.O.Box 1416, Minneapolis, MN 55440

Rorschach. In Exner, J.E. (1978). *The Rorschach: A comprehensive system* Vol. 2. New York: John Wiley & Sons.

Wechsler Adult Intelligence Scale—Revised (WAIS-R), by David Wechsler (1981). Available from Psychological Corporation, Harcourt Brace Jovanovich, 757 Third Avenue, New York, NY 10017.

Woodcock Reading Mastery Tests, by R.W. Woodcock (1973). Available from American Guidance Service, Inc., Publishers' Building, Circle Pines, MN 55014.

APPENDIX A

SSP Organizational Chart by Clinical Assignment

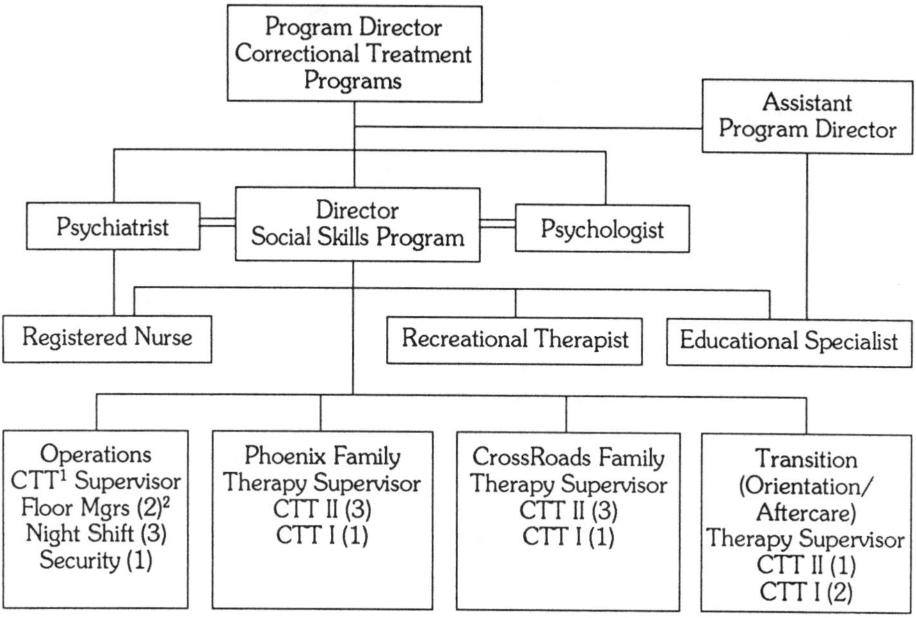

To maintain consistency and continuity of operational and clinical program goals, staff attend meetings as follows:

Daily: shift change (to transfer treatment information)

Semi-weekly: Treatment Team meetings (to discuss resident progress and to develop treatment plans)

Weekly:

- general staff meetings (to discuss program changes, concerns, treatment crises, and to provide staff inservice training)
- individual meeting by CTTs with their respective Therapy Supervisors for clinical supervision
- CTTs assigned to a particular group with the Therapy Supervisor to discuss group process and treatment-culture development
- Therapy Supervisors, Transition Therapist, Educational Specialist, CTT Supervisor, and the Recreational Therapist with the Director for administrative and/or clinical supervision
- CTTs with their Therapy Supervisors for clinical supervision in treatment provided in the behavioral laboratory

(continued)

[1] CTT = Correctional Treatment Therapist.

[2] Numbers in parentheses indicate staffing strength.

Bi-monthly: management meetings for the Director, Therapy Supervisors, Transition Therapist, CTT Supervisors, Registered Nurse, Educational Specialist, and Recreational Therapist

Or, to look at it another way, below is the meeting breakdown by staff position:

CTTs	**Supervisors**	**Treatment Team**[3]
<u>Daily</u>	<u>Daily</u>	<u>Semiweekly</u>
Shift change	Shift change	Treatment planning/ progress review
<u>Weekly</u>	<u>Weekly</u>	<u>Weekly</u>
Staff mtg.	Staff mtg.	Staff mtg.
Clinical Supervision	Clinical Supervision	
Family Group Culture	Family Group Culture clinical supervision	Administrative/clinical supervision[4]
Behavioral Therapy clinical supervision	Administrative/clinical supervision	
	Behavioral Therapy clinical supervision	
	<u>Bimonthly</u>	<u>Bimonthly</u>
	Management meeting	Management meeting[5]

[3] The Treatment Team is made up of the SSP's Director, Psychiatrist, Psychologist, Therapy Supervisors, Educational Specialist, Recreational Therapist, Registered Nurse, and Correctional Treatment Therapist (CTT).

[4] Supervisory personnel, the Educational Specialist, and Recreational Therapist only.

[5] All Treatment Team members except the Psychiatrist, Psychologist, and CTT.

APPENDIX B

SSP Treatment Schedule

	MONDAY	TUESDAY	WEDNESDAY	THURSDAY	FRIDAY	SATURDAY	SUNDAY
6:00 AM	Wake-Up						
7:00	Breakfast						
8:00	Housekeeping						
9:00	A.T.	A.T.	A.T./ Orientation	A.T.	A.T.	Breakfast	
10:00	Group P&C ****		Group (P)/ Workshop (C)		Group P&C		
11:00		Group Orientation				Housekeeping	
12:00 PM	Lunch						
1:00	School	Workshop (C)	School	Orientation Class	School		
2:00			Journal				
3:00	Workshop	Workshop	Workshop	Group (C)/ Workshop (P)	Group (C)/ Workshop (P)		
4:00	*	*		*	*		
5:00	Dinner						
6:00	Canteen	Group	** A.T.	Canteen ***	Journal	Journal	Journal
7:00	A.T.	SA Group		Group (P)	Community Activity	A.T.	AA Training
8:00	Journal		AA Group	Journal			
9:00	Television						
10:00	Lights Out						
11:00							
12:00							

Aftercare Treatment

Hours:
- * Debriefing 4:30 - 5:00 pm
- ** Tx Group 6:00 - 7:30 pm
- *** Support Group 6:00 - 7:30 pm
- **** Relapse Wksp. 10:00 - noon

Visiting Hours:
Tuesday 8:00 - 10:00 am
Wednesday 7:30 - 9:00 pm
Saturday 1:00 - 3:00 pm
Sunday 1:00 - 3:00 pm

A.T. Activity Therapy   P - Phoenix Family   C - Crossroads Family

APPENDIX C

SSP Developmental Change Model for Intellectually Disabled Sex Offenders

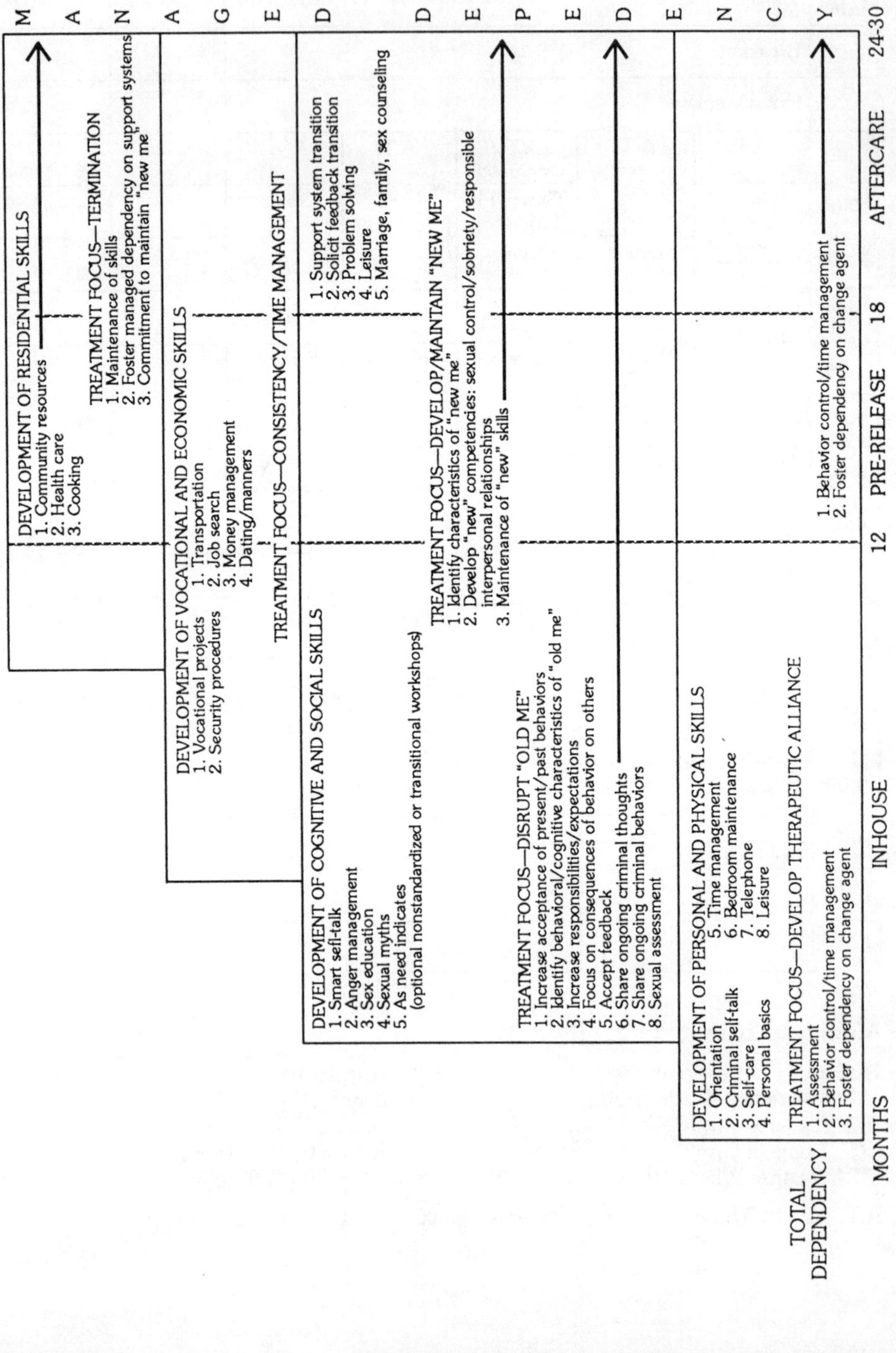

APPENDIX D

SSP Treatment Flow Chart

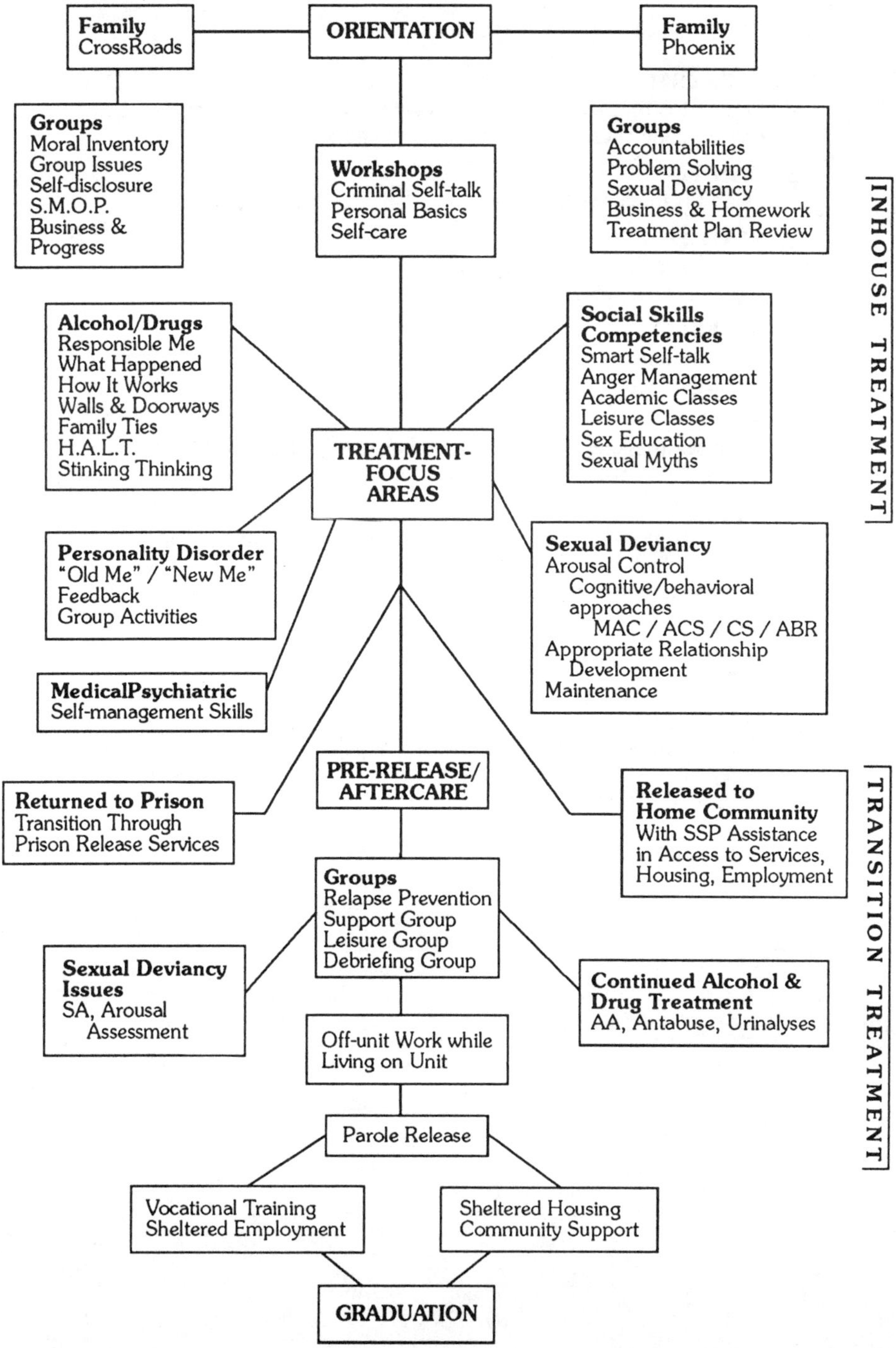

APPENDIX E

SSP Criminal Self-talk Statements

1. **LEFT OUT**
   Left Out is that feeling of being rejected, worthless, and empty. Left Out thinking says: "I'm willing to do anything to belong."
2. **CAN'T**
   I Can't is thinking: "I just can't do it. It's too hard, so I quit."
3. **SHUT DOWN**
   Shut Down is when the person thinks: "I won't say anything, I won't hear anything, I won't see anything, and I won't do anything."
4. **ME FIRST**
   Me First thinking says: "I am the best, I deserve the best, and everyone else is garbage."
5. **POOR ME**
   Poor Me thinking blames others when things don't go his way. He thinks: "It's not fair, it's someone else's fault."
6. **BULLY**
   The Bully thinks: "The only important thing is to get my way." The Bully thinks his needs and his rights are to be respected, but doesn't think about anyone else's needs or rights.
7. **NOW**
   NOW thinking says: "I want what I want, when I want it, and I want it NOW!"
8. **GOOD GUY**
   Good Guy thinking says: "I am really giving them what they want so I'm really not a bad guy. I'm a Good Guy." The way he thinks about his victims is: "They want it."

APPENDIX F

SSP Criminal Self-talk Worksheets

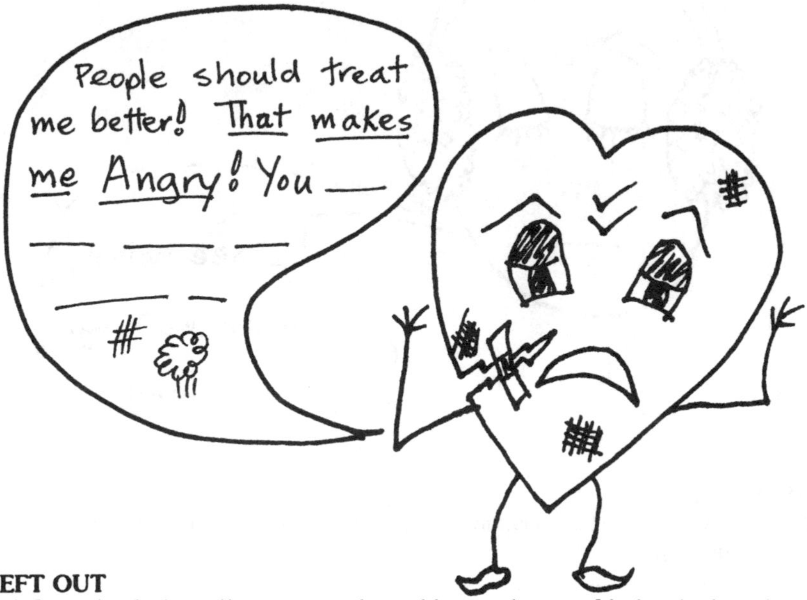

LEFT OUT

Left Out is that feeling of being rejected, worthless, and empty. It's that thinking that says: "I'm willing to do anything to belong."

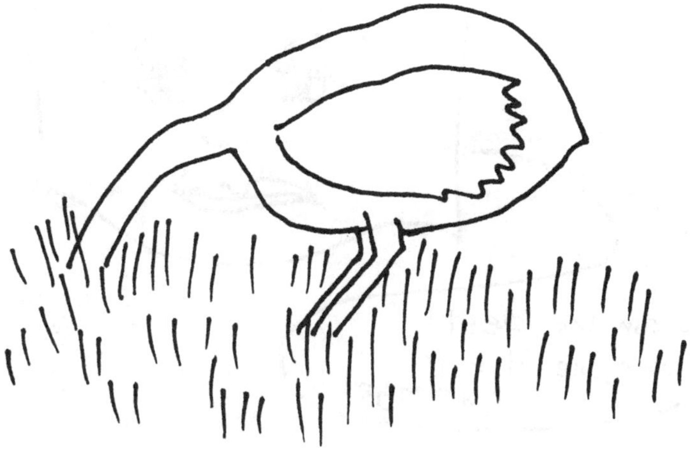

I CAN'T

I Can't happens when I have an attitude that says: "I just can't do it. It's too hard, so I quit."

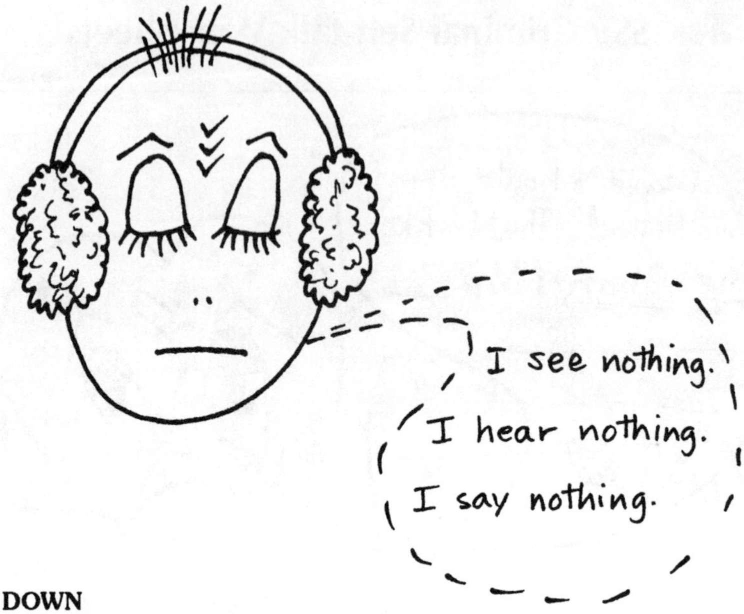

SHUT DOWN
Shut Down is when I won't say anything, I won't hear anything, I won't see anything, and I won't do anything.

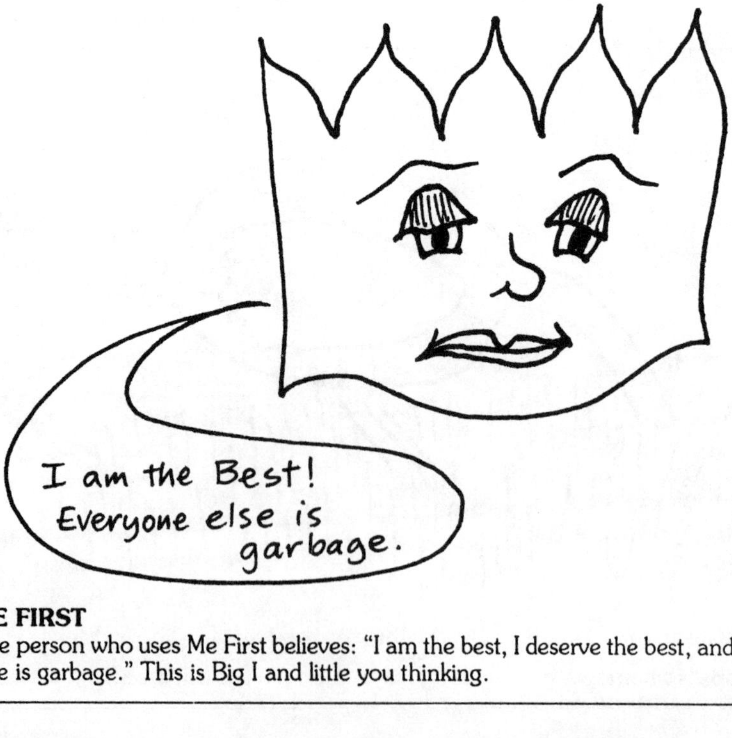

ME FIRST
The person who uses Me First believes: "I am the best, I deserve the best, and everyone else is garbage." This is Big I and little you thinking.

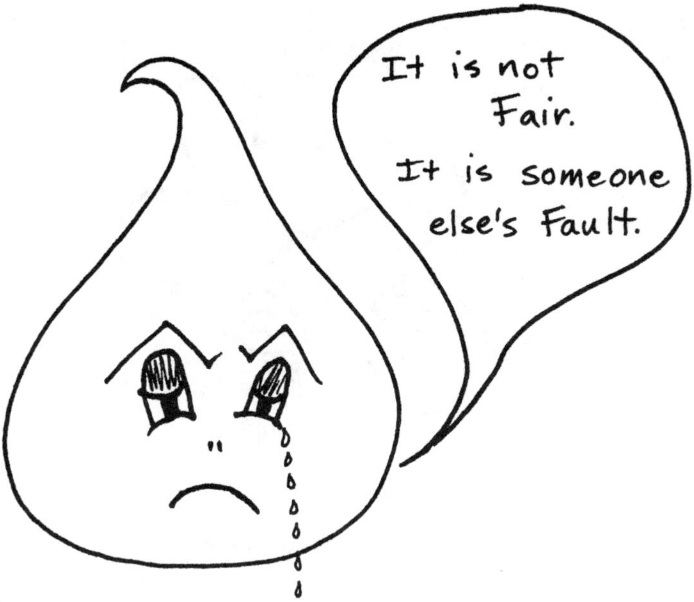

POOR ME
The person who uses Poor Me blames others when things don't go his way. He thinks: "It's not fair, it's someone else's fault."

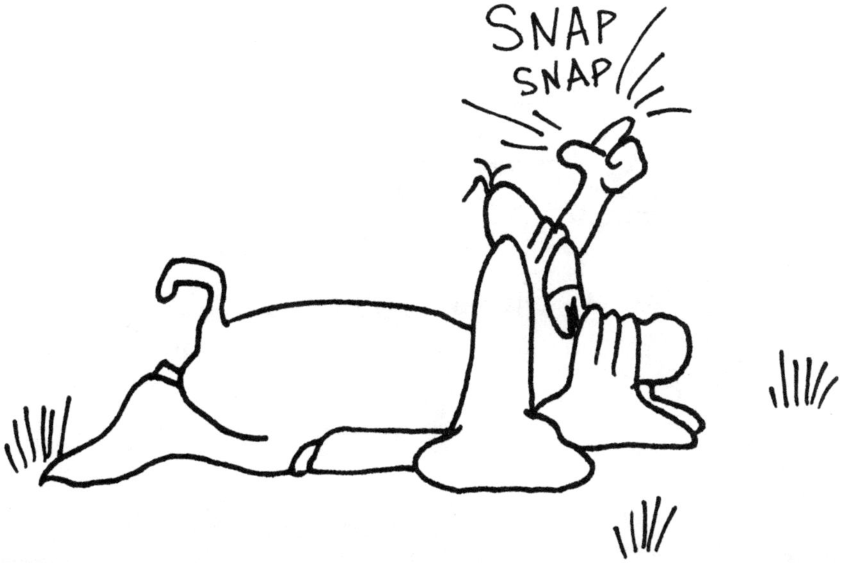

BULLY
The Bully tells himself: "The only important thing is to get my way." The Bully thinks about his needs and rights, but doesn't think about anyone else's needs or rights.

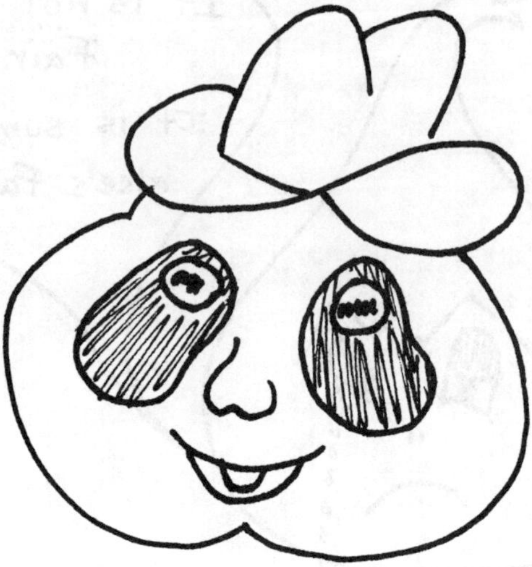

NOW
The person who uses Now thinking says to himself: "I want what I want when I want it and I want it NOW!"

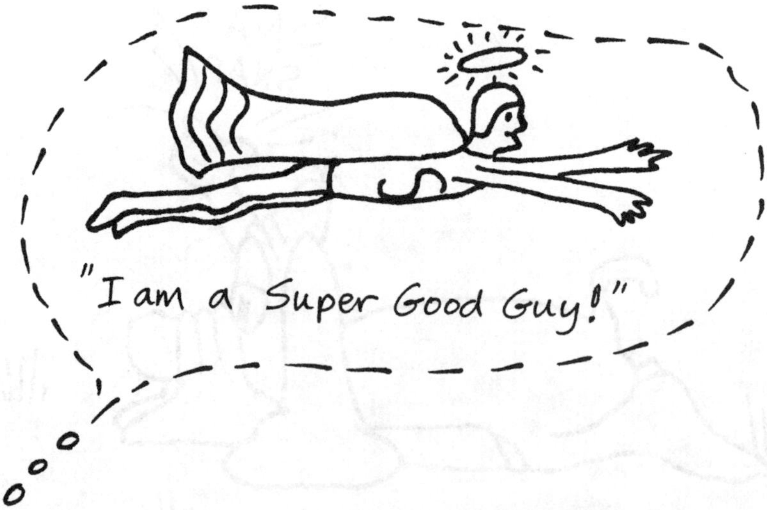

GOOD GUY
The person who uses Good Guy thinking says to himself: "They want it." The person using this kind of thinking tells himself that: "I am really giving them what they want so I'm not really a bad guy. I'm a Good Guy."

SSP Criminal Self-talk Test Sheets

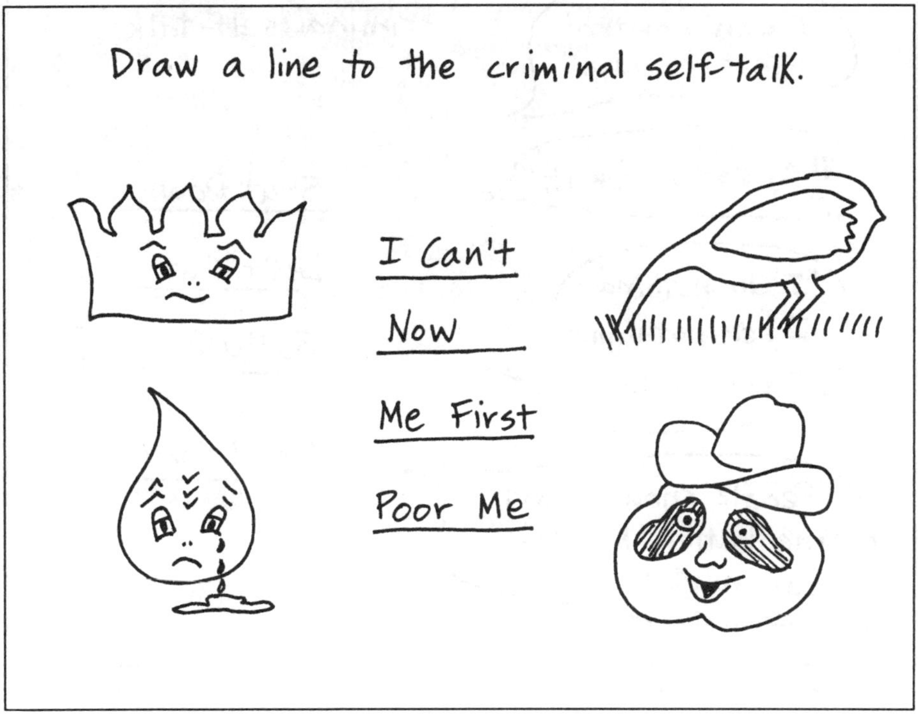

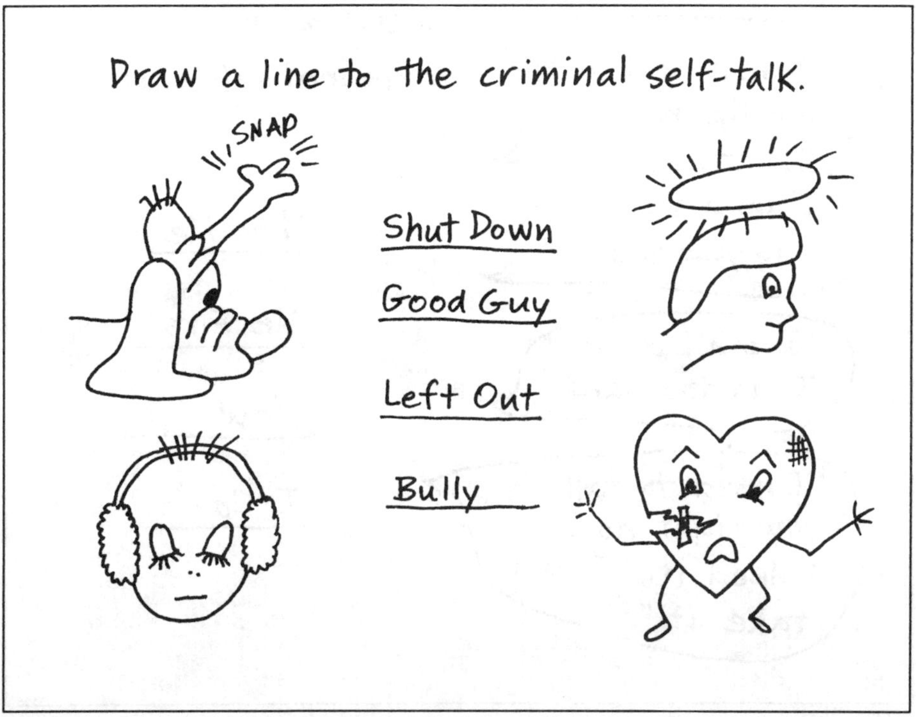

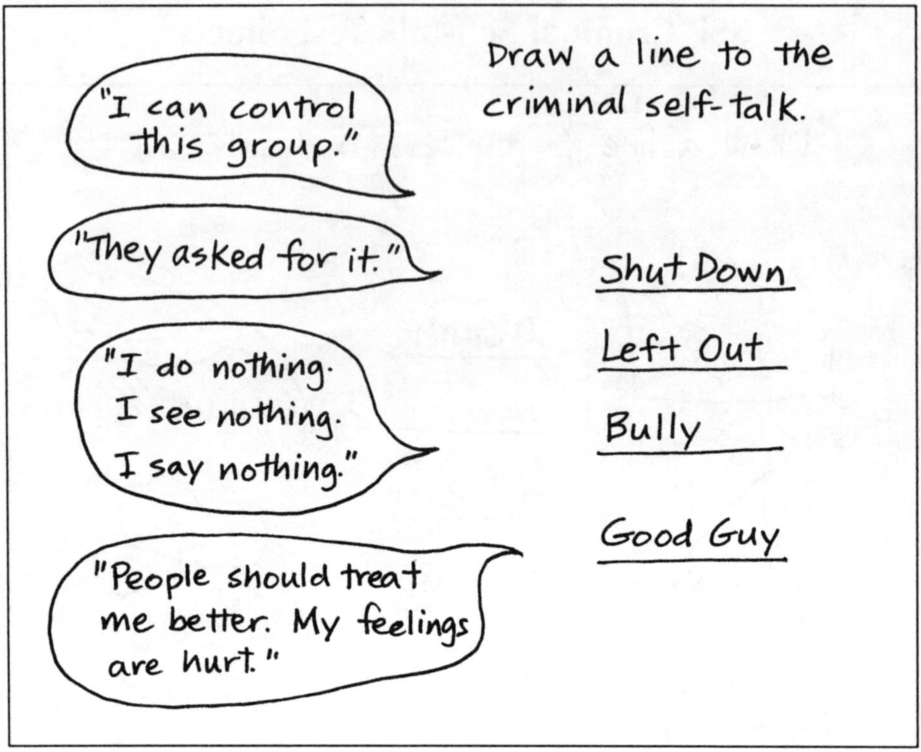
"I can control this group."
"They asked for it."
"I do nothing. I see nothing. I say nothing."
"People should treat me better. My feelings are hurt."
Draw a line to the criminal self-talk.
Shut Down
Left Out
Bully
Good Guy

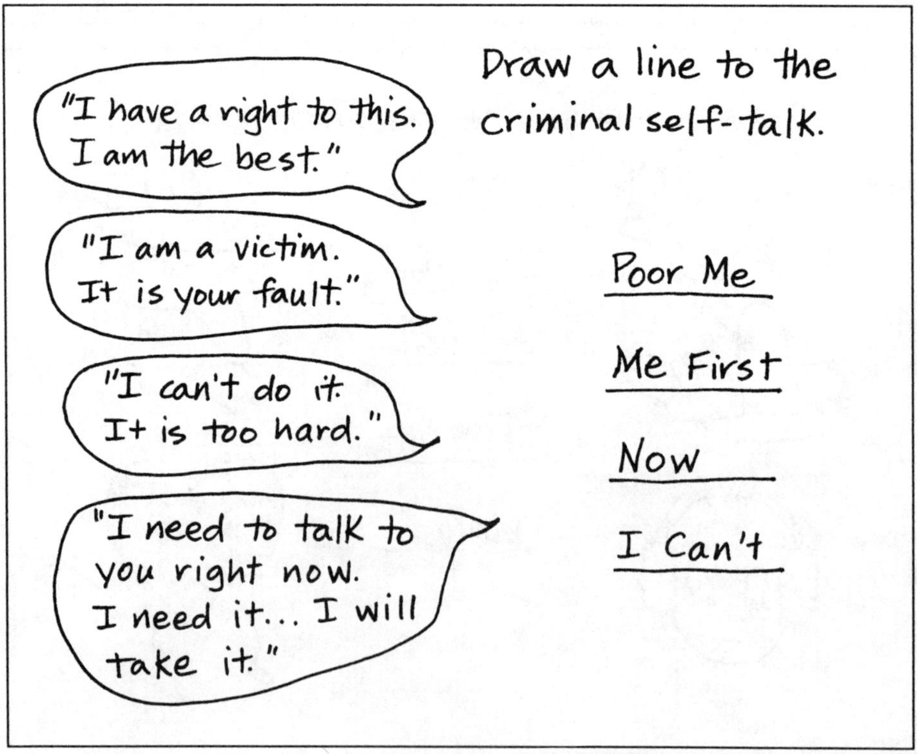
"I have a right to this. I am the best."
"I am a victim. It is your fault."
"I can't do it. It is too hard."
"I need to talk to you right now. I need it... I will take it."
Draw a line to the criminal self-talk.
Poor Me
Me First
Now
I Can't

APPENDIX G

SSP Self-care Worksheet

1. List four daily personal hygiene tasks:

   a. ______________________ c. ______________________

   b. ______________________ d. ______________________

2. List six hygiene products:

   a. ______________________ d. ______________________

   b. ______________________ e. ______________________

   c. ______________________ f. ______________________

3. How often do you change your clothes? ______________________

4. Why do people bathe? (Circle all correct answers.)
   a. Mom made me do it.
   b. To keep clean.
   c. To smell good.
   d. To lose weight.

5. Why do people need to brush their teeth? (Circle all correct answers.)
   a. To reduce breath odor.
   b. To keep from getting AIDS.
   c. To reduce tooth decay.
   d. To brush away plaque.

6. What is plaque? ______________________

7. How often should we visit the dentist? ______________________

8. When do you use deodorant? ______________________

9. Describe how you floss your teeth. ______________________

   ____

10. From the list below underline the ones that describe good self-care.

______ Safe sex	______ Eating fatty foods
______ Shampoo hair	______ Asking for help when needed
______ Wash without soap	______ Going to the dentist
______ Friendship	______ Saying "Thank you"
______ Eating vegetables and fruit	______ Poor posture
______ Clean clothes	______ Avoid too much sunshine
______ Saying "No"	______ Body odor
______ Exercise	______ Positive attitude
______ 3 hours of sleep at night	______ Hobbies
______ Expressing good feelings	______ Clean and trimmed hair

11. Write the word BAD in front of each bad self-care habit in the list above.

12. From the words listed above pick out one BAD self-care habit and explain why it will hurt you. ______________________

    ____

APPENDIX H

SSP Therapeutic Recreational Activities

Purpose

Therapeutic recreational activities in the Social Skills Program meet the following objectives:

- to increase *active and passive skills* in a wide variety of leisure activities;
- to increase *socialization skills* in leisure activity settings;
- to provide *prescriptive treatment intervention* for specific resident problem areas as needed;
- to provide *daily physical exercise* programming for all residents.

All SSP residents are in need of increased healthy leisure skills. The residents have physical and intellectual limitations that have caused developmental delays in their ability to provide themselves access to the rewards of healthy and responsible leisure involvement. Their lack of socialization skills is compounded by severe personality disorders, limiting their ability to bond and develop positive interpersonal relationships. Some treatment issues respond better to modalities using the specific expertise of the Recreational Therapist than to other treatment modalities. Finally, all residents need daily exercise because of the sedentary lifestyle encouraged by institutional living.

Services Provided

The following services are provided by the Activity Therapist and/or SSP staff:

1. *Structured classes* are taught to residents in a wide variety of leisure activity areas. Each hour-long class is held once or twice a week for six weeks. Seven to ten different structured classes are offered to clients each term.[6]
2. *Specific activities* are designed to address individual residents' treatment issues needing attention beyond general program objectives.
3. *Holiday activities,* parties, and special events are organized.
4. A *weekly group meeting* is held for Pre-release/Aftercare residents to develop leisure skill activities through discussion, planning, and community trips.
5. *Equipment and access to instruction* are made available to help residents develop leisure activities during their scheduled free-choice activity period.

Assessment of Resident Needs

Therapeutic recreational needs of residents in the SSP are identified in three ways:

1. All new residents are identified as having two primary needs: to increase active and passive leisure skills, and to increase socialization skills in leisure settings. Every specific structured activity is designed to meet the residents' program objectives.
2. Within 45 days of admission, each resident is evaluated by the Recreational Therapist, who completes a Therapeutic Recreational Assessment focusing on

---

[6] A partial list of classes and activities offered in 1989 includes: Jazzerobics, Sign Language, Mask Making, Current Events, New Games, Drama, Volleyball, Soccer, Ping Pong, Soccer, Mime, Video, Horseshoes, Croquet, Studio Arts, and card and board games such as Pictionary, Dominoes, and Yahtzee.

the resident's strengths and weaknesses in the two primary need areas. Any other needs identified in the assessment process by observations, interview, and the Leisure Barriers Test[7] are outlined in the Therapeutic Recreational Assessment for review by the interdisciplinary Treatment Team.

3. Any other needs of the resident are identified in the Treatment Team process, using information and observations of Team members.

Delivery System

In order to provide the most services for residents, SSP unit staff conduct therapeutic recreational activities under the supervision of the Recreational Therapist.

A minimum of seven structured activity classes—held mornings and evenings—are scheduled for each six-week term. One week before the term starts, class offerings are posted; each resident selects his top two choices. With the goal of creating a group dynamic that motivates and involves the residents, the Recreational Therapist assigns residents to classes based on their needs and preferences.

The Recreational Therapist has a minimum of five resident-contact hours in conducting classes each week. The Recreational Therapist assigns other structured classes to SSP staff based on their skills and interests. Staff are responsible for designing course content, outlining lesson plans, and implementing these classes. At the end of each six-week term, a two-week break period allows staff to document residents' treatment progress as measured by the objectives outlined in their lesson plans.

Since therapeutic recreational activities are integrated into the entire treatment milieu, any resident who develops new treatment issues during recreational classes is referred to his CTT for help in processing them with his treatment group.

As a member of the interdisciplinary Treatment Team, the Recreational Therapist presents the client's treatment progress relative to the program-defined objectives and shares any other needs or problems that may have been observed.

The Recreational Therapist meets weekly with Pre-release/Aftercare residents as a group to plan leisure activities in the community, to discuss each resident's individual leisure plans, to take community trips, and to process problems that have developed.

With staff assistance, the Recreational Therapist organizes and implements holiday activities and special events as prescribed by the SSP Treatment Team.

Supervision

The Recreational Therapist supervises staff in designing and implementing all structured recreational classes, including observing classes and meeting with staff individually as needed. The Recreational Therapist provides any training and instruction needed by staff in facilitating activity classes.

The Program Director meets weekly with the Recreational Therapist to review whether therapeutic recreational activity objectives are being met.

Documentation

The Recreational Therapist completes a comprehensive Therapeutic Recreational Assessment on each resident within 45 days of admission and writes a treatment plan and progress summary on each resident at least every 90 days.

Staff members write a progress note on each resident—reviewed by the Recreational Therapist—at the completion of their class.

---

[7] See Resources.

APPENDIX I

SSP Alcohol/Drugs Worksheet

Do I See Who I Really Am?

I. What are my handicaps: (What do I see about myself?)

A. Physically:

B. Socially:

C. Educationally:

D. Emotionally:

E. In Relationships:

F. Growth:

G. Other Areas:

II. What feedback did my CTT have to add?

APPENDIX J

The Power Pendulum

This diagram demonstrates the swift process of gaining and losing power:

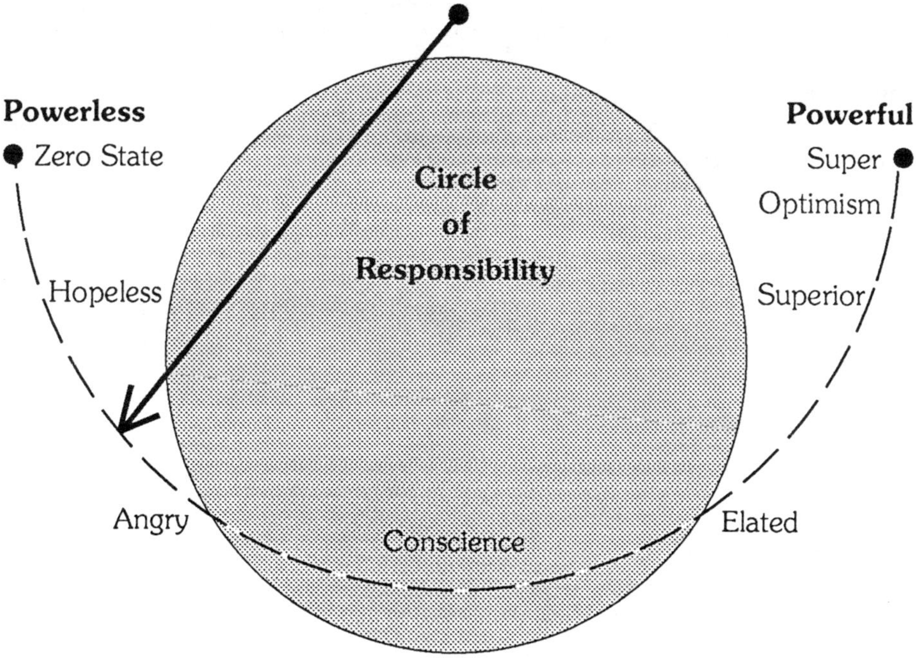

Criminals almost never center themselves in the circle of responsibility. Criminals want to be at the powerful side of the pendulum swing. But they don't maintain the high due to forces acting on them that push them toward powerlessness.

Kim Conner, Oregon Correctional
Treatment Program

APPENDIX K

SSP Sexual Arousal Assessment Informed Consent

A Sexual Arousal Assessment is done to help your therapist and the Treatment Team learn more about your sexual urges. If you choose to do this, you will be assessed in the Behavioral Therapy Lab (BT room). You will place a small rubber gauge around your penis while in a room alone. This will measure how hard you get while you watch sexual slides and videos and listen to tapes. You will see and hear "good" sex and "bad" sex descriptions.

Benefits

The main benefit will be that your true sexual urges will be known by your BT and you. A plan can then be written to treat the problems that are found. This will not be shared with the Parole Board without your O.K.

Risks

There are certain risks involved. You may feel anxious, uncomfortable, depressed, nervous, or angry. You may worry so much about how you will do that you may have problems getting hard during or after the assessment. If you have any of these problems, a BT will help you, if you ask.

Other Methods

Other ways of assessing you are interviews and written tests. You might choose these if you feel that the BT work would cause you major health or mental problems.

Choosing Treatment

This assessment is not required. You will not be sent back to prison for refusing to do BT work. A BT assessment must be approved by the Treatment Team before you can do it.

Permission

I have reviewed this form with my BT and understand the benefits and risks. I know that I can ask questions, slow down, or quit at any time.

____

Resident Signature Date

____

Staff Witness Date

APPENDIX L

SSP Sexual Arousal Assessment Raw Data Sheet

Client Name:______________________ Behavioral Therapist:__________

Date:________________ Purpose:______________________________

Stimuli Material:____

	Type	MM	%	EST.[8]	COMMENTS
1.					
2.					
3.					
4.					
5.					
6.					
7.					
8.					
9.					
10.					
11.					
12.					
13.					
14.					
15.					
16.					
17.					
18.					
19.					
20.					

[8] Client's estimate of his arousal.

APPENDIX M

SSP Sexual Arousal Assessment Raw Data Summaries

Client Name ______________________________

Dates of Lab Sessions ______________________________

Videos

1. __________ _____ ______________________________
2. __________ _____ ______________________________
3. __________ _____ ______________________________
4. __________ _____ ______________________________

Type % COMMENTS

Slides

	FA	FC	FYC	MA	MC	MYC[9]
High						
Avge.						
Low						
#						

Audiotapes

	FAM	FCM	FAR	FCR	MAM	MCM	MAR	MCR[10]
High								
Avge.								
Low								
#								

Other

1. Self Fantasies _____ ______________________________
2. __________ _____ ______________________________
3. __________ _____ ______________________________
4. __________ _____ ______________________________

Type % COMMENTS

---

[9] Female Adult, Female Child, Female Young Child, Male Adult, Male Child, Male Young Child.

[10] These are the same gender and age categories as above (minus the "Young Child" age group) with the addition of a force dynamic: Mutual or Rape.

APPENDIX N

SSP Sexual Arousal Assessment

Client Name ______________________________ B.T. ______________________________
Hospital # ______________________________ Date ______________________________

Purpose of Assessment:

Observations:

Conclusions:

Recommendations:

APPENDIX O

SSP Cognitive/Behavioral Interventions Informed Consent Forms

APPENDIX O-1

SSP Minimal Arousal Conditioning Informed Consent

APPENDIX O-2

SSP Covert Sensitization Informed Consent

APPENDIX O-3

SSP Assisted Covert Sensitization Informed Consent

APPENDIX O-4

SSP Aversive Behavioral Rehearsal Informed Consent

APPENDIX O-1

SSP Minimal Arousal Conditioning Informed Consent

Minimal Arousal Conditioning (MAC) is done so that you can learn to stop your penis from getting hard to bad sex thoughts.

How It Works

This is how it works:

1. You will tell your Behavioral Therapist (BT) about a time when you had bad sex. This will be the time you think about most. Your BT will write about that in a lot of detail.

2. You will learn to tell the story into a tape recorder. When your penis begins to feel hard, you will stop and smell ammonia to make your penis soft again. Then you will start the story over. You will do this for 30 minutes each day.

3. Once or twice a week you will go into the lab with your BT. There you will tell the story with a gauge on your penis. Your BT will be able to tell you when to smell the ammonia. You will learn when your penis gets even a little hard.

Benefits

The main benefit is that you will learn how to stop your penis from getting hard to bad sex thoughts. This could help you stop yourself from doing a sex crime.

Risks

MAC has some risks. You may become nervous, depressed, angry or have sexual problems for a while after doing this treatment. You could even feel like hurting yourself. These feelings could carry over to the way you get along with others on the unit. These will not likely last for a long period of time. If you have any of these problems, your BT will be able to help you, if you ask.

Other Methods

Other ways to teach you how to control bad sex thoughts offered by the Social Skills Program include group therapy and one-to-one counseling. The risks of these methods are the same as MAC.

Choosing Treatment

This treatment is advised but not required. You will not be sent back to prison for refusing to do MAC. MAC must be approved by the Treatment Team before you can do it. You may quit MAC at any time.

Permission

I have reviewed this form with my BT and understand the benefits and risks. I know that I can ask questions, slow down, or quit at any time.

____

Resident's Signature Date

____

BT's Signature Date

APPENDIX O-2

SSP Covert Sensitization Informed Consent

Covert Sensitization (CS) is done to teach you how to stop thinking about bad sex. It also teaches you what to do instead.

How It Works

This is how it works:

1. You talk into a tape recorder about a time that led to having bad sex.
2. Before you get to the part about the bad sex, you yell loudly "STOP!!"
3. You then use your STOP self-talk such as, "It's not worth it, I don't need it."
4. Now you use your GO self-talk such as "I need to go to the Unit" or "I need to talk to my sponsor."
5. Then you say all the bad things that can happen to you if you have bad sex again.
6. You say this whole thing over and over again for 30 minutes every day.
7. After that you give your tape to your BT. Your BT can answer any questions and can help you get used to doing these tapes.

Benefits

The main benefit is that you will be able to learn to stop bad sex thoughts before it is too late. You will learn what to do so you won't do another sex crime. You will be able to recall the bad things that could happen to you if you did do another sex crime.

Risks

CS has some risks. You may become nervous, depressed, angry, or have sexual problems while doing this treatment. You could even feel like hurting yourself. These feelings could carry over to the way you get along with others on the unit. These will not likely last for long periods of time. If you have any of these problems, your BT will be able to help you, if you ask.

Other Methods

Other ways to teach you how to control bad sex thoughts offered by the Social Skills Program include group therapy and one-to-one counseling. The risks of these methods are the same as CS.

Choosing Treatment

This treatment is advised but not required. You will not be sent back to prison for refusing to do CS. CS must be approved by the Treatment Team before you can do it. You may quit CS at any time.

Permission

I have reviewed this form with my BT and understand the benefits and risks. I know that I can ask questions, slow down, or quit at any time.

____

Resident's Signature Date

____

BT's Signature Date

APPENDIX O-3

SSP Assisted Covert Sensitization Informed Consent

Assisted Covert Sensitization (ACS) is done to teach you a way to control your bad sex thoughts. First, it teaches you things that can happen to you from bad sex. Second, it teaches you how to think good sex thoughts instead.

How It Works

This is how it works: Your Behavioral Therapist (BT) will teach you how to make an ACS tape. It will have four parts:

1. A relaxation part.
2. A short "bad sex" part.
3. The results of "bad sex."
4. A "good sex" part.

These tapes will last at least 15 minutes. You will make them every day and turn them in to your BT.

After you learn to make the tapes right, you will train yourself in the lab to stop bad sex thoughts by smelling bad odors. You will train yourself outside of the lab by snapping a rubber band on your wrist when you have bad sex thoughts. You will also train yourself by only thinking of good sex thoughts when you masturbate.

This treatment should take from 6 to 8 weeks. You may ask for some follow-up sessions after this treatment is complete.

Benefits

The main benefit is that you may be able to learn to stop your bad sex thoughts and replace them with good sex thoughts. This could help you stop doing sex crimes. It will also help you think about the bad things that could happen if you commit another sex crime.

Risks

ACS has some risks. You may become nervous, depressed, angry, or have sexual problems while doing this treatment. You could even feel like hurting yourself. These feelings could carry over to the way you get along with others on the unit. These will not likely last for a long period of time. If you have any of these problems, your BT will be able to help you, if you ask.

Other Methods

Other ways to teach you how to control bad sex thoughts offered by the Social Skills Program include group therapy and one-to-one counseling. The risks of these methods are the same as ACS.

Choosing Treatment

This treatment is advised but not required. You will not be sent back to prison for refusing to do ACS. ACS must be approved by the Treatment Team before you can do it. You may quit ACS at any time.

Permission

I have reviewed this form with my BT and understand the benefits and risks. I know that I can ask questions, slow down, or quit at any time.

____

Resident's Signature　　　　　　　　　　Date

____

BT's Signature　　　　　　　　　　Date

APPENDIX O-4

SSP Aversive Behavioral Rehearsal Informed Consent

Aversive Behavioral Rehearsal (ABR) is done for two reasons. First, it helps you change how you think and feel about having sex with children. It will help you feel bad about it. Second, it gives your therapist a lot of information about how you do sex crimes.

How It Works

This is how it works: First you make a videotape of yourself while you pretend to do a sex crime. You use a dummy that looks like your victim. You act out exactly what you did. While doing this, you say your thoughts and feelings. This videotape is first seen by just you and your therapist. When you are ready, it is shared with the group and other staff. The staff and the group may ask questions and may say their feelings about the crime.

Benefits

The main benefit of ABR is that you may be able to stop bad sex thoughts. You will likely recall your ABR when you think of having sex with children. This will help you to stop yourself from hurting another child.

There are two other benefits. First, you will know more about how you commit sex crimes. This may help you to stop before you go too far. Second, you will be able to share your pattern with others. This will allow them to better help you.

Risks

ABR has some risks. You may be upset for a few weeks. Some have become very depressed for even longer. You may even feel like hurting yourself. Some have become very angry and quit all treatment. You might have trouble getting a "hard on" or "coming" for a while after ABR.

This treatment could cause you problems with staff and residents. They may feel and act differently as they learn more facts about your crime.

If you have ever tried to hurt yourself, let your therapist know now. If you have ever heard voices when no one was there, tell your therapist now.

If you have any of these problems while doing ABR, the Social Skills Program staff will be there to help you.

Other Methods

There are not many other ways that work as well as ABR. The other ways to change how you think and feel about having sex with children are:

1. Being confronted by a former victim who is now an adult.
2. Smelling bad odors in the BT room while you think of having sex with children.
3. Being shocked in the leg or arm in the BT room when you think of sex with children.
4. Sharing all the little details of your crime with close members of your family.

All these methods have the same risks as ABR.

Choosing Treatment

This treatment is not required. You will not be sent back to prison for refusing to do ABR. ABR must be approved by the Treatment Team before you can do it. You may quit ABR at any time.

Permission

I have looked over this form with my therapist and understand the benefits and risks of ABR. I know that I can ask questions, slow down, or quit at any time.

____

Resident's Signature Date

____

BT's Signature Date

APPENDIX P

SSP Transition Application (Pre-release)

Resident's Name ______________________________ Date ____________

Marital Status ______________________________ Release Date ______

A. Deviant sexual outlet when I have problems:

1. Sexual ______________________________

____

____

2. Money ______________________________

____

3. Job ______________________________

____

____

4. Social ______________________________

____

____

5. Drugs/Alcohol ______________________________

____

____

B. What are my personal strengths? ______________________________

____

____

C. What kind of help am I going to need as I plan to leave the Inhouse group?

____

____

____

____

____

D. What kind of help am I going to need when I move into the community?

____

____

____

____

Group's Approval ______________________________

____

Therapist Approval ______________________________

APPENDIX Q

SSP Transition Checklist

____________________________ ______________ ______________

NAME OSH # PAROLE DATE

10 months prior ____________________ (date)

_____ Begin application for transition to be okayed by TS(i) and Inhouse group, and to be filed in discharge section of chart by 9 months prior.

9 months prior ____________________ (date)

_____ MMPI

_____ Begin Relapse Workshop

_____ Medium custody in place

_____ Treatment Team meets to outline transition plan, after full review of inpatient treatment progress and methods since admission. TS(i) dictates for eventual use in discharge summary.

_____ Request minimum custody

8 months prior ____________________ (date)

_____ Begin leisure groups, daily debriefings, workshops as offered.

_____ Completion of all Inhouse required treatment, to include: ____major BT work; ____relapse/behavior pattern; ____living sober plan; ____arousal control contract; ____other ____________________.

_____ Maintain Inhouse schedule except when scheduled into transition activities. Accountability is to Inhouse group and privilege board. Off-unit passes are initialed first by CTT and signed by TS (a).

_____ Meet with AT to develop leisure contract. Place in chart, in Discharge section under Assessments.

7 months prior ____________________ (date)

_____ Begin Aftercare groups

_____ Evaluation for Antabuse complete and in chart

_____ Begin on-grounds minimum custody passes with peers

_____ CTT arranges on-grounds worksite

6 months prior ____________________ (date)

_____ Accountability switches to transition group, no longer on Inhouse privilege board. CTT continues to write and supervise treatment plan, working with TS(i) and TS(a).[11]

_____ Begin half-time on-grounds work experience, arranged and monitored by CTT.

---

[11] Therapy Supervisor (Inhouse) and Therapy Supervisor (Aftercare).

NAME ______ OSH # ______ PAROLE DATE ______

- ______ Begin off-grounds treatment related passes with peers.
- ______ Begin weekly schedule and budget with transition staff.
- ______ Develop job search goals and plan with CTT and/or transition staff. Place in chart, under Assessments in Discharge section.
- ______ SRF[12]/group home application in
- ______ Renew release of information form

5 to 4 months prior ______________ (date)

- ______ May attend week-long job search seminar
- ______ May begin job search "practice" per guidelines

4 to 3 months prior ______________ (date)

- ______ Begin intensive job search, per guidelines
- ______ Begin off-grounds leisure passes with peers
- ______ Formal meeting with client and Inhouse and transition staff

3 months prior ______________ (date)

- ______ Complete physical exam
- ______ MMPI
- ______ Repeat sexual assessment filed under Assessments in Discharge section of chart.
- ______ Discharge contract complete and in chart
- ______ Treatment Team outlines discharge direction, special parole conditions, and level of supervision.
- ______ Start work at SRF if appropriate
- ______ Research and attend leisure activities with peers
- ______ Move into transition cottage, if appropriate, when employed.
- ______ Write Parole Board
- ______ Begin one-to-one's with TS(a).

1 month prior ______________ (date)

- ______ SSI application if appropriate
- ______ Discharge Treatment Team. Invite all participating agencies. Finalize logistical plan and outline treatment direction. Send copies of Treatment Team review to all cooperating agencies.
- ______ Resident to meet with parole officer
- ______ Arrange release subsidy money with Release Services

This checklist is filed in the Discharge section of the chart.

[12] SRF is the Salem Rehabilitation Facility.

APPENDIX R

Relapse Prevention
Cognitive/Behavioral Model of Reoffense

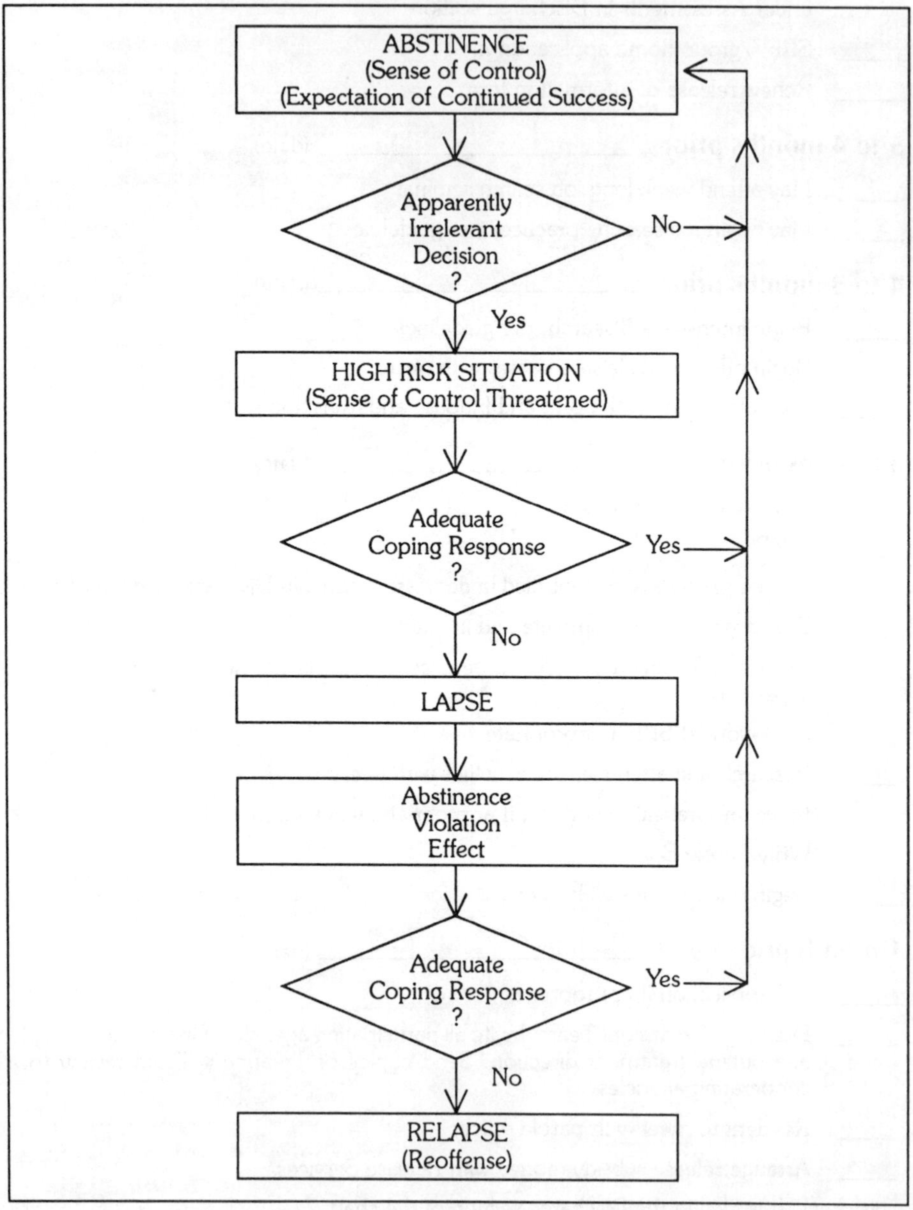

Adapted from Pithers, W.D., Kashima, K.M., Cumming, G.F., Beal, L.S., & Buell, M.M. (1988). Relapse prevention of sexual aggression. In R.A. Prentky & V.R. Quinsey (Eds.). *Human sexual aggression: Current perspectives* (p. 248). Annals of the New York Academy of Sciences Vol. 528. New York: The New York Academy of Sciences. Used by permission.

APPENDIX S

SSP Discharge Contract

Resident's Name____________________ Date________________

Marital Status____________________ Release Date____________

A. Behavior Pattern (attached)

B. Employment ____________________

C. Social Commitments ____________________

D. Recreational Interests ____________________

E. Special Conditions ____________________

F. Budget/Transportation ____________________

G. Living Situation ____________________

Continued Therapy Plan ____________________

Resident's Signature____________________

Aftercare Therapist's Signature ____________________

Parole Officer's Signature ____________________

Review Dates ________________ ________________

Resident Aftercare Therapist

Other Safer Society Publications

Pathways: A Guided Workbook for Youth Beginning Treatment by T. Kahn, 1990, $15.00

Who Am I and Why Am I in Treatment? A Guided Workbook for Clients in Evaluation & Beginning Treatment by R. Freeman-Longo & L. Bays, 1988, 80 pages, $10.95

Why Did I Do It Again? Understanding My Cycle of Problem Behaviors by L. Bays & R. Freeman-Longo, 1989, 80 pages, $10.95

How Can I Stop? Breaking My Deviant Cycle by L. Bays, R. Freeman-Longo, & D. Hildebran, 1990, 80 pages, $10.95

Fuel on the Fire: An Inquiry into "Pornography" & Sexual Aggression in a Free Society by J. Rosenberg, 1989, 96 pages, $13.95

Female Sexual Offenders: An Exploratory Study by R. Mathews, J. Matthews, & K. Speltz, 1989, 112 pages, $17.50

Adults Molested as Children: A Survivor's Manual for Women & Men by E. Bear with P. Dimock, 1988, 76 pages, $12.95

A Model Residential Juvenile Sex Offender Treatment Program: The Hennepin County Home School by J.W. Heinz, S. Gargaro, & K.G. Kelly, 1987, 144 pages, $23.00

Treating the Young Male Victim of Sexual Assault: Issues and Intervention Strategies by E. Porter, 1986, 96 pages, $12.50

Retraining Adult Sex Offenders: Methods & Models by F.H. Knopp, 1984, 319 pages, $20.00